Mosby
Dedicated to Publishing Excellence

Editor: Linda L. Duncan
Developmental Editor: Jo Salway
Project Manager: John Rogers
Sr. Production Editor: Kathleen L. Teal
Electronic Production Coordinator: Chris Robinson
Design Coordinator: Renée Duenow
Cover Illustration: April Goodman Willy
Manufacturing Supervisor: Kathy Grone

Printed in the United States of America
Composition by Mosby Electronic Production, St. Louis
Printing/binding by R.R. Donnelley & Sons Company

Mosby–Year Book, Inc.
11830 Westline Industrial Drive
St. Louis, Missouri 63146

International Standard Book Number: 0-8016-8065-4

95 96 97 98 99 / 9 8 7 6 5 4 3 2 1

Mosby's Fundamentals of
VETERINARY TECHNOLOGY

Veterinary Clinical Laboratory Procedures

Margi Sirois, M.S., R.V.T.

Veterinary Technology Program
Camden County College
Blackwood, NJ

with 66 *illustrations*
and 24 *color plates*

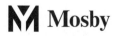 Mosby

St. Louis   Baltimore   Berlin   Boston   Carlsbad   Chicago   London   Madrid
Naples   New York   Philadelphia   Sydney   Tokyo   Toronto

Mosby's Fundamentals of
VETERINARY TECHNOLOGY

Veterinary Clinical
Laboratory Procedures

For Dale, Jennifer, and Daniel

Preface

This book is intended as a textbook for clinical hematology, clinical chemistry, and urinalysis courses taught in veterinary technology programs. I have assumed a basic knowledge of anatomy, physiology, and biochemistry, but have included reviews of these areas with most of the chapters. Every effort has been made to present this material at a level which is appropriate for the student of veterinary technology.

Vast technological advances in the clinical laboratory field have contributed to an expanded role for the practicing veterinary technician. The veterinary technician is often responsible for developing and maintaining an in-house clinical laboratory which is both cost-efficient and reliable. This responsibility requires an extensive knowledge of basic laboratory procedures, as well as an understanding of the biochemical principles involved in clinical laboratory testing. A knowledge of these parameters for both manual and automated laboratory procedures is essential. Textbooks which are available for veterinary medical students and medical laboratory technology students generally contain only small parts of the information needed by the veterinary technology student, or are written at a level which is beyond the scope of the technicians training. I have attempted to gather this material in one volume while limiting the scope of the material to that required of a graduate veterinary technician employed in either clinical practice, research, or in the veterinary reference laboratory. Although the primary focus of this text is canine and feline testing, references to exotics and large animals have been included as often as practical.

ACKNOWLEDGEMENT

This book would not have been possible without the support and guidance of my friends, colleagues, and students at Camden County College. I am especially grateful to Professor Marianne McGurk of Camden County College and Dr. Doug McBride of LaGuardia Community College for their advice. Special thanks to Dr. Harriet Doolittle for her encouragement and to graduate veterinary technicians Tim Lasslett, Tracey D'Imperio, and Jayne Wilcox for sharing their opinions and helping to prepare the illustrations for this text. I am indebted to the staff at Mosby, and in particular to Jo Salway for her patience.

Margi Sirois

Contents

Glossary, 141

Laboratory instrumentation and equipment

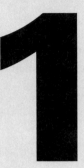

PERFORMANCE OBJECTIVES
After completion of this chapter, the student will:

Identify commonly used laboratory instruments and equipment.

Describe proper procedures for operation, care,
and maintenance of clinical laboratory equipment.

Identify commonly used laboratory pipettes.

Choose correct pipettes for various laboratory tests.

Describe the principle behind spectrophotometric analyses.

Explain the procedures for one point calibration and standard curve construction.

Describe the principle behind the impedance method of particle counting.

Differentiate between precision and accuracy.

List the common sources of error in clinical testing.

Define the terms "control" and "standard"
and explain the use of each in clinical laboratory testing.

T he veterinary technician plays a vital role in medical management of diseased animals. In small animal practice, the technician's ability to quickly provide reliable clinical laboratory data can have a major impact on the smooth operation of the veterinary clinic. In recent years, the development of a variety of types of inexpensive analytical equipment has simplified the operation of an in-house clinical laboratory. In some veterinary practices, clinical laboratory tests are sent to outside reference and commercial laboratories. The use of outside laboratories eliminates the need for a large variety of specialized equipment, but increases the amount of time before the clinician receives laboratory data. Frequently, the data are necessary to provide confirmation of a diagnosis before treatment can be started. This delay can have detrimental effects on patient health. In any case, the technician must be familiar with the various test methodologies employed by any commercial laboratory. Many commercial laboratories are designed primarily to assay human samples and often the laboratory personnel are unfamiliar with the variations in test results when animal samples are run.

LAB DESIGN

The veterinary clinical pathology laboratory should be located in an area separate from other hospital operations. Alternatively, a corner of a room can be dedicated for clinical testing. The area should be well lit and contain a sink. It must also be large enough for adequate counter space to accomodate instrumentation and provide a comfortable work area. Sensitive equipment, such as cell counters and spectrophotometers, should not be located adjacent to centrifuges or water baths. Drawers or cabinets located beneath or above the laboratory counter are necessary to store related equipment and supplies. A refrigerator with a small freezer compartment is also required. Electrical outlets must be conveniently located and in adequate numbers to ensure an uncluttered work area. Some equipment may also require the use of an electrical surge protector.

LABORATORY MEASUREMENT AND MATHEMATICS

Accurate laboratory measurements and data reporting require a thorough knowledge of the metric system. Metric system units for the expression of weight, length, and volume are the gram, meter, and liter, respectively. Prefixes are used with these basic units to denote fractions or multiples of a unit. For example, the prefix 'milli-' means one thousandth of a part. A milligram, therefore, is one thousandth of a gram and a milliliter is one thousandth of a liter. A summary of the more commonly used prefixes and their abbreviations is found in Table 1-1.

In an effort to standardize data reporting, it is recommended that laboratory data be reported in SI units. SI, or Système Internationale, uses metric system notation with specific designations for measurement of certain laboratory parameters. For example, in SI units, wavelength is designated in nanometers and blood albumin concentration in grams/liter. In veterinary medicine, the transition to SI units is not yet complete. A number of references may still be found which use conventional units.

Dilutions

The veterinary technician is frequently required to prepare dilutions of substances such as reagents, standards, and patient samples. Concentrations of dilutions are often expressed as ratios of the original volume to the new volume. For example, if 10μl of patient sample is combined with distilled water to yield a total new volume of 100μl, then the dilution ratio is 10:100. This reduces mathematically to 1:10. Results of any clinical testing on that diluted sample would then be multiplied by 10 to provide the actual test result for the undiluted sample. This type of dilution is frequently used when an assay result is above the capabilities of the test methodology employed.

Dilutions of standard solutions are also needed for construction of standard curves for use in clinical chemistry analyses. A standard is a nonbiological solution of a particular component and contains a known concentration of that component. Several dilutions of the standard are made and each dilution is then read in the spectrophotometer. For example, if a standard solution of bilirubin contains 20 mg/dl and serial dilutions of 1:5, 1:10, and 1:20 are made, then the concentration of these dilutions is 4 mg/dl, 2 mg/dl, and 1 mg/dl, respectively. These concentrations are then used when plotting the standard curve.

INSTRUMENTATION AND EQUIPMENT

The microscope

The foundation of any clinical laboratory is a good quality binocular compound light microscope (Fig. 1-1). The mechanical features of the microscope may vary depending on

TABLE 1-1

Metric system prefixes

Prefix	Abbreviation	Definition
femto	f	10^{-15}
pico	p	10^{-12}
nano	n	10^{-9}
micro	μ	10^{-6}
milli	m	10^{-3}
centi	c	10^{-2}
deci	d	10^{-1}

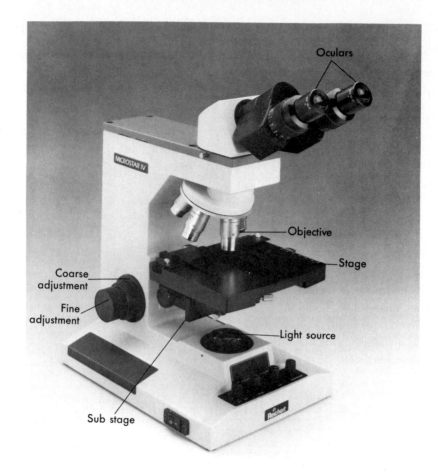

Fig. 1-1. Typical binocular microscope for clinical laboratory procedures. (Courtesy of Leica, Inc., 111 Deer Lake Rd., Deerfield, IL 60015.)

the size of the laboratory and the type of testing that will be performed. Ideally, the microscope used for examination of fecal and urine specimens will be separate from that used for hematologic analysis.

All compound light microscopes utilize three sets of lenses to produce an enlarged two-dimensional image of a specimen. Light is focused through the object with the condenser lens. The objective lens receives this light and generates an enlarged image which is magnified further at the eyepiece or ocular lens. A clinical microscope usually has four objective lenses in a rotating base. The actual magnification of these lenses may vary depending on the manufacturer of the microscope and the particular needs of the laboratory. The lenses typically used are 4× (scanning), 10× (low power), 45× (high power), 100× (oil immersion). Most clinical microscopes employ a 10× ocular lens. The exact magnification of each lens is etched on the side of the lens. To determine total magnification, multiply the individual magnifications of the ocular and objective lenses. Therefore, a 100× oil immersion lens is capable of enlarging an image by one thousand.

Both the magnification and the resolving power should be considered when choosing a microscope. Resolving power is the ability of the microscope to distinguish fine detail. This is a function of the wavelength of light used and the numerical aperture (size of the opening) of the objective. A resolving power of between 0.1μ and 0.2μ is adequate for the general purpose clinical laboratory. It is usually not necessary to incur the additional expense of a microscope with higher resolution unless the laboratory is involved in research.

Additional features which should be considered are the field of view of the eyepiece and the type of objective lenses. Most clinical microscopes are supplied with wide-field eyepieces and these provide the best overall image. Planachromatic lenses provide a flat field image, with the entire field of view in focus. Microscopes with achromatic lenses may have some blurring of the specimen toward the outer edges of the field. A mechanical stage is also an essential feature, allowing for accurate positioning of an object. Phase contrast and/or darkfield illumination may be required in some laboratories.

A microscope is a precision instrument that must be properly maintained. The microscope manufacturer provides complete care and use guidelines with each instrument. In general, cleanliness of the optical components is of prime importance. All lenses should be wiped clean with lens tissue at least daily. The oil immersion lens must be cleaned of oil after each use. Should oil buildup occur, a small amount of xylene on lens tissue will help to remove it. Excess use of xylene is discouraged as this can damage the objective.

Centrifuge

A centrifuge is an essential component of the clinical laboratory; it is designed to facilitate separation of substances of different densities that are in solution. All veterinary practice laboratories require at least one centrifuge. A microhematocrit centrifuge is designed to hold capillary tubes while a clinical centrifuge can hold test tubes. Some centrifuges combine both of these capabilities (Fig. 1-2).

There are a great number of clinical centrifuges available. The most common type contains an angled head. Tubes are placed within holders which are at a fixed angle within the centrifuge head. One disadvantage of this type is that they are generally designed for only a single-size tube. Smaller volume tubes require the use of adaptors. This is not a concern with the swinging arm type centrifuge, which can usually accomodate varying size tubes. Regardless of the type of centrifuge used, care should be taken that the tubes are oriented properly within the centrifuge, that the centrifuge is properly balanced, and that the lid is securely fastened. Tubes should be placed with their open ends toward the center of the instrument and counterbalanced with tubes of equal size and weight. This will ensure that no liquid is forced out of the tubes during centrifugation. An improperly balanced centrifuge will wobble and can result in tube breakage or damage to bearings. Should a tube break inside the centrifuge, it must be dismantled and the broken glass carefully and thoroughly removed. Likewise, any spilled liquid should be promptly and thoroughly removed. The use of a disinfectant may also be required.

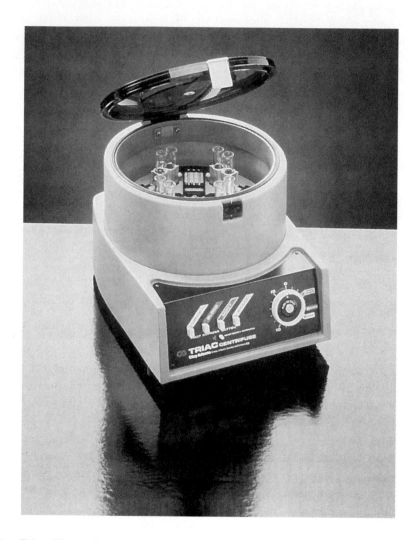

Fig. 1-2. Triac Clinical Centrifuge. This model can be used for both microhematocrit determinations and centrifugation of blood and urine specimens. (Photo courtesy of Becton-Dickinson Co. Primary Care Diagnostics, 7 Loveton Circle, Sparks, MD 21152.)

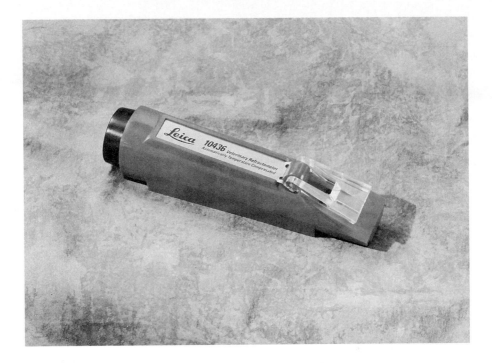

Fig. 1-3. The refractometer is used for determination of urine specific gravity and total plasma protein. (Photo courtesy of Leica Inc., 111 Deer Lake Road, Deerfield, IL 60015.)

Centrifuges are usually calibrated in RPMs times 1000. Thus, a dial setting of 2 is actually 2000 RPMs. The relative centrifugal force can be calculated with the equation: $RCF = 1.118 \times 10^{-5} \times r \times RPM^2$, where r = the radius in centimeters from the center of the centrifuge head to the axis of rotation. RCF is normally expressed as gravity or G force. Many centrifuges also contain timers which will automatically turn the equipment off after a preselected time has elapsed. Always wait until the centrifuge comes to a complete stop before beginning to remove items. The brake found on some models should be used only in cases of equipment malfunction when the centrifuge must be stopped quickly. As part of the periodic routine laboratory maintenance procedures, the carbon brushes in the centrifuge should be checked. Periodic verification that the centrifuge is attaining the desired speed is done with a tachometer.

Refractometer

The refractometer is a device used to measure the refractive index of a solution. Refractive index is defined as the degree that light is bent when it is passed through a liquid, and is a function of the amount and type of solid material dissolved in the liquid. In clinical practice, this instrument is calibrated to give direct readings of total protein in serum samples and specific gravity of a urine sample (Fig. 1-3).

The zero setting on the instrument should be checked with distilled water on a regular basis and adjusted as necessary. Since the refractometer is an optical instrument, care must be taken to ensure that the optical surfaces are properly maintained.

Pipettes

There are literally thousands of different pipettes and pipetting devices available for use in the clinical laboratory. The specific ones chosen will depend on the particular applications needed. In general, there are three main types: transfer, graduated, and automatic.

Transfer pipettes are designed to hold or transfer liquids when critical volume measurements are not necessary. They are commonly made of plastic but may be made of glass. Some are available which can deliver material dropwise. The Pasteur pipette is an example of a transfer pipette.

Graduated pipettes may contain multiple gradations or have a single gradation. The latter are referred to as volumetric pipettes and are the most accurate of all measuring pipettes. They are usually calibrated as "to deliver" and are designated with "TD" at the top of the pipette (Fig. 1-4). This means that they are designed to deliver the specific volume of liquid. A small amount of liquid will remain in the tip of the pipette which must not be blown out. Microliter pipettes are volumetric and designed to measure very small volumes of liquid. These are calibrated as "TC" or "to contain" and always require rinsing with a diluent. The small amount of liquid remaining in the tip is blown out after rinsing.

The most commonly used multigraduated pipettes are the Mohr measuring pipette and the serological pipette. The Mohr is available in a wide range of sizes and is the most accurate of the multigraduated pipettes. It is calibrated as "TD" and some liquid may remain in the tip of the pipette, which is not dispensed. Serological pipettes are less accurate and are usually calibrated as "TD with blow-out." The volume of liquid remaining in the tip must be blown out. TD blow-out pipettes are identified with a double etched or frosted band at the top of the pipette.

The pipette chosen should always be the most accurate one available for a particular application. If a multigraduated pipette is to be used, the one which measures closest to the needed volume will be the most accurate. For accurate measurement, liquids must be at room temperature. Several types of pipetting devices are available, the simplest of which is a rubber bulb. More elaborate devices such as pumps can also be used or aspirator tubing can be attached to the end of the pipette. Never pipette any liquid by placing your mouth directly on the pipette!

Automatic pipettes are available in a wide variety of sizes and types, some which measure single volumes only and others which have variable volume settings.

SPECTROPHOTOMETER

The spectrophotometer is designed to measure the amount of light which is transmitted and/or absorbed by a solution. There are a great number of models available, all with the same basic principle (Fig. 1-5). Light is passed through a device which fragments the light into equally dispersed segments. The desired wavelength of light is chosen either with a filter or a wavelength cam and then passes through the sample. The light that is transmitted through the sample reaches a photodetector, is amplified, and converted to electrical energy. This electrical energy then reaches a meter or readout device. The units given at the meter or readout device may be in percent transmittance, percent absorbance, and/or concentration units depending on the particular model and configuration of the instrument.

The spectrophotometer may employ either a flow-through cell to draw the solution into the light path or have a well to accommodate a cuvette. Although similar in appearance, a test tube is not an acceptable substitute for a cuvette. Cuvettes are optical instruments, composed of either glass or plastic and require special handling to achieve accurate results. Avoid touching the sides of the cuvette. If necessary, polish the outside of the cuvette with lens tissue to remove any fingerprints. Disposable polystyrene cuvettes tend to be more costly while glass cuvettes require additional handling procedures which may be time consuming. They must be scrupulously cleaned with nonabrasive cleansers and properly matched. Cuvettes obtained from a single manufacturer are matched by filling each about ¾ full with distilled water. Place the first cuvette in the sample well and set the instrument to read about midrange transmittance (the actual number does not matter). Place each remaining cuvette in the well and record the percent transmittance of each. Use only those cuvettes within 1% of each other.

The spectrophotometer passes a specific wavelength of light through the sample. The wavelength chosen is usually that which will give maximum absorbance of the light by the sample. For example, a substance appears blue-green because light within the red portion of the spectrum is absorbed and blue-green light is transmitted. If light within the red portion of the spectrum was selectively passed through the same sample, essentially all the light would be absorbed and none would be transmitted. This sample would have maximal absorbance in the red area of the spectrum, and therefore a wavelength in that range would be chosen. The instrument is set to read zero absorbance, utilizing a cuvette with distilled water as a blank. In some cases, a reagent blank is required to eliminate the effect of the reagent color.

In order for a specific substance to be accurately quantified in the spectrophotometer, the relationship between absorbance, percent transmittance, and concentration must fol-

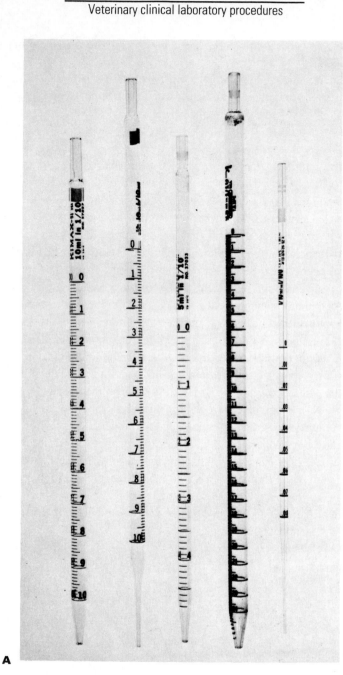

Fig. 1-4. Examples of TD pipettes. (From Kaplan LA, Pesce AJ: *Clinical Chemistry: Theory, Analysis, and Correlation*, ed 2, 1983, St. Louis, Mosby.)

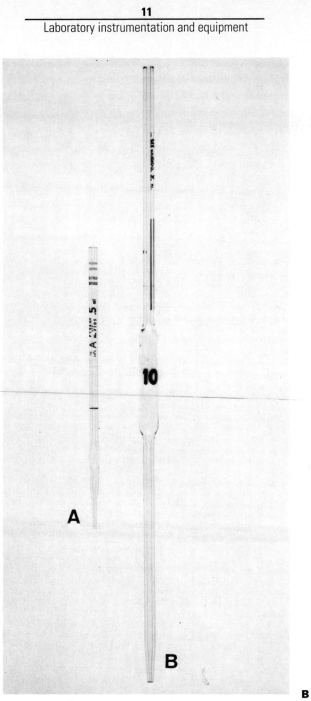

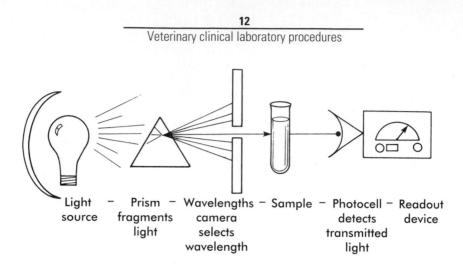

Light – Prism – Wavelengths – Sample – Photocell – Readout
source fragments   camera   detects   device
        light   selects   transmitted
                    wavelength   light

Fig. 1-5. The principle of spectrophotometry. A tungsten light source is commonly used for visible wavelengths.

low Beer's law. Beer's law states that the concentration of molecules of a colored substance is directly related to the amount of monochromatic light absorbed by the substance and inversely and logarithmically related to the amount of light transmitted. Absorbance may also be referred to as the optical density of a substance. The analysis must follow Beer's law over the entire range of standards used. Concentration can then be determined by either a one point calibration or from a standard curve.

The one point calibration requires analysis of a standard solution of the substance each time a patient sample is tested. The concentration of the substance in the patient sample is then calculated as follows:

$$\text{Concentration of patient sample} = \frac{(\text{Absorbance of sample} \times \text{concentration of standard})}{\text{absorbance of standard}}$$

A standard curve is sometimes preferred to the one point calibration. It is necessary to analyze standards only once to prepare the curve. Serial dilutions of the standard are prepared and the absorbance and percent transmittance of each dilution is determined at the wavelength of maximum absorbance. The concentration of each dilution is graphed against the absorbance on straight line graph paper (Fig. 1-6). Percent transmittance versus concentration is plotted on semilogarithmic paper. The concentration of any subsequent patient sample is determined by measuring its absorbance and/or percent transmittance and reading the corresponding concentration from the standard curve. Each time a new batch or lot number of reagents, or a new instrument is used, a new standard curve must

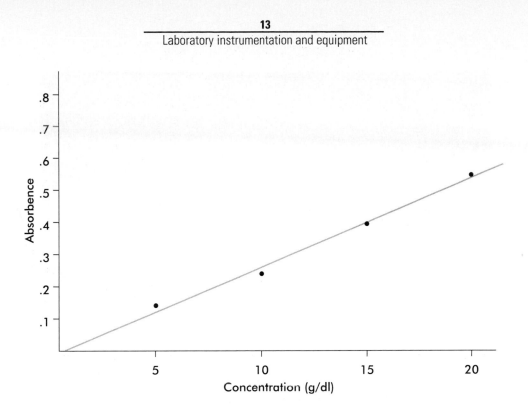

Fig. 1-6. Completed standard curve for hemoglobin plotting absorbance vs. concentration.

be prepared. The standard curve is specific for the lot number of reagent, as well as the specific instrument and equipment used.

AUTOMATED ANALYZERS

A number of different analyzer types are available for the veterinary hospital laboratory. Hematology analyzers are reasonably priced and are capable of performing up to seven hematologic tests on each patient sample. The majority of these instruments work by measuring the number of all particles of a specific size as they pass through an aperture. This requires that the technician be familiar with the sizes of the various cellular components for each species seen at the particular practice. Chemistry analyzers are also affordable and offer greatly reduced assay times. These analyzers are similar in principle to the spectrophotometer. Some employ sets of filters to select the desired wavelength. Several also utilize "dry" reagent systems, which greatly reduces the storage space needed for laboratory supplies (Fig. 1-7).

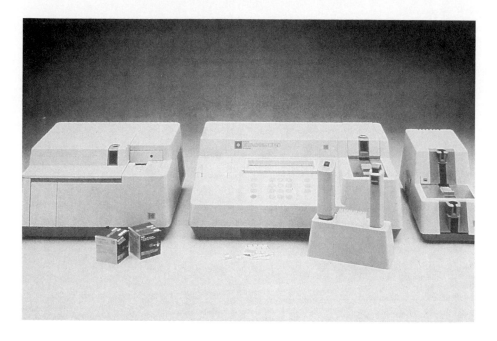

Fig. 1-7. The Kodak DT60 Analyzer with modules for testing of additional chemical parameters and electrolytes. (Reprinted courtesy Eastman Kodak Co.)

The Coulter Counter is a commonly used instrument for hematology testing. This instrument utilizes what is referred to as the electrical impedance method to quantify the number of particles in a sample. The particles can be of any size or type. In hematology, this instrument is used to count blood cells. An electrolyte solution is used to dilute the sample. The solution is drawn through an aperture which has a weak electric current running through it. As cells of a particular size pass through the aperture, a specific volume of the electrolyte solution is displaced. This causes a change in the resistance in the path of the electrical current flow. The number of changes within a specific period of time is directly proportional to the number of cells suspended in the electrolyte solution (Fig. 1-8). To utilize the electrical impedance method, the technician must be familiar with the size of the cellular elements of a particular species. The instrument counts only particles of a specific size. To obtain valid data, the technician must set the instrument for the cell sizes characteristic of the species being tested.

A number of types of hematology analyzers have recently been marketed to the veterinary practitioner. Many of these utilize an electrical impedance method. Others are available which use optical methods with a focused laser beam to count particles. In some cases, these instruments may provide only an estimate of the cell count.

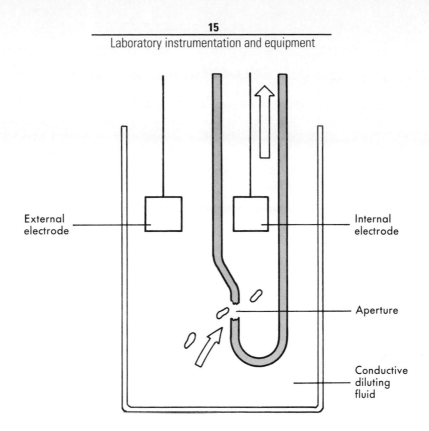

External
electrode

Internal
electrode

Aperture

Conductive
diluting
fluid

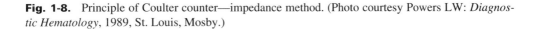

Fig. 1-8. Principle of Coulter counter—impedance method. (Photo courtesy Powers LW: *Diagnostic Hematology*, 1989, St. Louis, Mosby.)

MISCELLANEOUS EQUIPMENT

For certain clinical chemistry analyses and some coagulation studies, a water bath capable of maintaining a constant temperature of 37° Centrigade may be required. The temperature of the bath should be checked frequently.

Although not an essential part of the small veterinary practice laboratory, a slide dryer is a welcome addition to the busy hematology laboratory. The dryer can significantly reduce the time spent waiting for slides to air dry and can improve the quality of stained smears.

For the high-volume laboratory, an aliquot mixer is necessary to ensure that all samples and control materials remain thoroughly mixed while awaiting assay procedures.

LABORATORY SAFETY

Laboratory safety is an integral part of laboratory procedures. The veterinary clinical laboratory must have an established method for ensuring that employees are properly trained in

Lab safety policy

The safety procedures contained in this document are designed to minimize any potential source of injury to employees of this facility. All employees are required to adhere to these policies to ensure a safe workplace for everyone.

The clinical lab is equipped with the following safety equipment: fume hood, eye wash station, electrical surge and drop-out extensions, first aid kit, pipettors, chemical spill cleanup kit, fire extinguisher, and fire blanket.

All employees are required to familiarize themselves with these devices and be able to use and operate them effectively.

General rules

1. Smoking, eating, or drinking is prohibited in the lab.
2. No foods or beverages may be stored in the lab refrigerator or general lab area.
3. Lab coats must be worn at all times.
4. Long hair must be confined while in the lab.
5. Shoes must be worn in the lab; open toe or canvas shoes are prohibited.
6. No pipetting of materials by mouth!
7. All employees are responsible for safe and proper operation of equipment. Read the operator's manual and be familiar with the operation of any instrument before attempting its use.

Laboratory housekeeping

1. All glassware must be washed immediately after use. Cracked or chipped glassware must be discarded at once.
2. All work surfaces must be cleaned with a 10% bleach solution at the end of the work period.
3. Lab work areas must be kept clear of personal belongings.
4. Employees must wash hands thoroughly before leaving the lab.

Reagents

1. Fume hood must be used for dispensing reagents with potentially hazardous fumes.
2. All reagents will be stored properly in designated areas.
3. Carrying reagents must be done cautiously, using unbreakable containers whenever possible.
4. All reagent, stock, and dispensing containers MUST be labeled with identity, date, and initials of individual preparing reagent and MUST contain proper hazard warning labels.

Biologicals

1. All biologicals (blood, urine, body fluid, control materials) must be treated as potentially infectious.
2. Disposable latex gloves MUST be worn at all times when handling or transporting biological materials.
3. Spilled biological material must be cleaned up with 10% bleach solution.

Disposal

1. Reagents suitable for sewage disposal should be poured into running water in the sink.
2. Hazardous reagents will be disposed of in proper central waste containers.
3. All reagent bottles must be thoroughly rinsed before disposal.
4. Biological materials and their containers should be disposed of in biohazard bags.

safe laboratory practices. The Occupational Safety and Health Administration (OSHA) mandates specific laboratory practices which must be incorporated into the lab safety policy of the veterinary practice. This should include care and maintenance of safety equipment such as eyewash stations and fire extinguishers. Laboratory safety policies should be in writing and maintained in an accesible location within the laboratory. Proper cleaning procedures for laboratory glassware and counter tops and use and disposal of hazardous and biological materials should be included. A sample of a lab safety policy is found in the box on p. 16.

QUALITY CONTROL

Specific quality control procedures are developed for each laboratory based on the number and types of tests performed. Even the smallest veterinary practice laboratory requires a program of quality control to ensure precise and accurate results. Accuracy refers to how a test value approximates its true value. Precision is a reflection of the reproducibility of a test method. Even the best technique and the highest quality of reagents will produce slight variation in test results. Errors in assay procedures can result from a number of sources, including improper use of glassware, instruments, or reagents, as well as use of inappropriate test methodologies and/or technician error (see box below). A rigorous quality control program can minimize the magnitude of these errors. Veterinary practices which utilize commercial laboratories should be familiar with quality control procedures at these locations. This is particularly important if the commercial laboratory is primarily involved in testing human specimens. Some techniques used for assay of human pathology specimens may be inaccurate when used for nonhuman samples.

Test selection

The test methodology chosen should always be the most precise and accurate one available for measurement of the particular constituent. A variety of professional organizations evaluate test methodologies for use in human medicine. Many of the tests used in veterinary

---

Common sources of error in the clinical lab

1. Inappropriate test conditions (temp, pH)
2. Poor quality reagents
3. Interfering substances in sample (lipemia, hemolysis, etc.)
4. Improper use of cuvettes (dirty, scratched, unmatched, etc.)
5. Stray light entering instrument
6. Fluctuating electrical power (power surges, light source fatigue, etc.)
7. Improper use of pipettes

medicine were developed for human use and have been adapted to animal systems. The Veterinary Laboratory Association reviews test methodologies for veterinary use. In some cases, a less accurate test may be preferred due to equipment availability and/or time constraints. Regardless of methodology, care must be taken that all procedures are strictly followed. A test that is designed to be performed at a particular temperature or pH may give inaccurate results if performed at a slightly different temperature or pH. Similarly, many tests require that reagents be added at timed intervals. Strict adherence to these timed sequences is crucial to achieving reliable results.

The technician must be familiar with the principle of all tests performed in the laboratory. This familiarity must include awareness of the limitations of a particular test, as well as substances that may interfere with the test. Test limitations may become important when measuring parameters at the upper and lower limits of the sensitivity of a test. For example, if a test is sensitive to a chemical constituent found in blood at levels between ten and forty mg/dl, a patient value that is above or below those levels may not be properly quantified. The presence of interfering substances in the sample will also affect the reliability of test results. Some anticoagulants interfere with test methodologies. Certain drugs given to the patient will also affect test results, frequently by inhibiting the test reaction. Photometric assays will be affected by any substance which increases the color development of a sample. Such substances include excess lipid material in the sample (lipemia). Lipemic samples are common when the animal has not been fasted prior to blood collection. Lysis of erythrocytes (hemolysis) may result when a sample has been improperly collected or may be the result of a pathologic condition. Analyses which rely on color development in the sample will be affected by lipemia or hemolysis. A serum blank is used in these cases to allow the operator to deduct the effect of hemolysis or lipemia from the optical density of the final reaction mixture. Commercial products are also available which clear lipid material from serum prior to assaying the sample.

Instrumentation & equipment

The types of equipment required for a test procedure will vary, but steps must be taken to ensure the correct equipment is chosen and that all equipment is working properly. The most accurate and well-maintained equipment will not correct for errors in technique. The technician must adhere to strict procedures in the use of any equipment. For example, a 10µl fixed-volume automatic pipette can be a highly accurate and precise measuring device. However, if the pipette is held at an angle, or the wrong size disposable tip is chosen, the device will not measure accurately. In addition, periodic checks on the calibration of this device are required. In time, an automatic pipette can develop barely perceptible defects in sealing gaskets which can greatly alter the volume measurement. All clinical laboratory equipment must undergo regular maintenance and calibration procedures. Verification that water baths reach and maintain a desired temperature, that centrifuges are reaching the desired RPMs, and that the spectrophotometer is providing the desired wavelength are cru-

cial to ensuring reliable results. The laboratory must have a schedule of periodic maintenance and calibration procedure for all equipment and maintain records of these procedures.

Analysis of control material

Controls are biological materials which contain specific quantities of blood or sera constituents. These are commercially available or may be prepared in-house by the technician.
Commercial controls are provided either assayed or unassayed and are available in both
normal and abnormal ranges of values. Assayed controls are supplied with a range of
expected values for each constituent present. Unassayed controls are generally less expensive, but each laboratory is responsible for determining the concentration of the constituents in the material. Preparation of controls in-house is accomplished by collecting and
pooling excess specimens. Preparation of pooled controls requires a greater investment of
time by the technician but reduces the total cost of running the laboratory. The excess samples should be organized by type of anticoagulant and type of abnormality before pooling.
For example, plasma samples taken utilizing sodium citrate anticoagulant from clinically
normal animals can be combined to yield a pool of citrated plasma control. As with commercially available unassayed controls, the laboratory is responsible for developing the
range of expected values for pooled control materials.

Regardless of source, the control should be analyzed each time an assay is performed on
a patient sample or batch of samples. The control is treated as if it were a patient sample.
Control results obtained are compared with those supplied by the manufacturer of the control material or the results expected from the in-house pool of control. A separate log of control data should be maintained in order to identify any trends in quality control, such as with
gradual deterioration in reagents over time (Fig. 1-9). It is helpful to graph control data on a

Quality Control Log

Date	Control ID Mfg	Lot #	Absorbance	%T	Concentration	Assay value	Comments	Technician

Fig. 1-9. Quality control log.

daily basis to visualize any potential problems (Fig. 1-10). Whenever control results do not agree with expected values, the entire procedure should be carefully analyzed to determine the source of error. Once the error is corrected, the patient samples from the batch of testing must be reassayed before results are reported to the clinician.

Training of laboratory personnel

A large variety of in-house instruments are marketed for use in veterinary practice which have greatly simplified test procedures. Although these instruments appear simple to use, proper training is vital to providing accurate results. The veterinary technician must ensure that all laboratory personnel are familiar with proper operation of equipment, as well as potential sources of error. As with all laboratory equipment, improper maintenance and poor technique can invalidate test results.

Continuing education of laboratory personnel is also crucial to good quality control. Since laboratory medicine is a rapidly changing field, measures to keep personnel well-informed are essential.

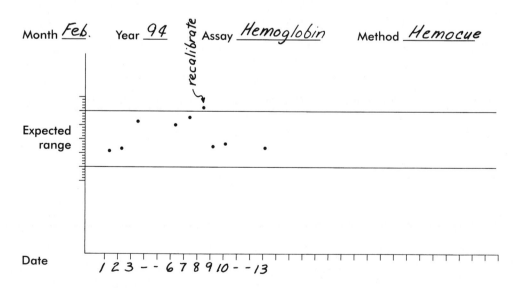

Fig. 1-10. Example of one type of daily control data graph.

KEY POINTS

1. Proper care and maintenance of laboratory equipment is essential for smooth operation of the laboratory and generation of reliable results.

2. Laboratory data should be reported in SI units.

3. Selection of and proper use of the correct pipette is crucial to the accuracy of test results.

4. The spectrophotometer is a precision instrument designed to measure the amount of monochromatic light which is absorbed by or transmitted through a substance.

5. Most automatic blood chemistry analyzers utilize the principle of spectrophotometry.

6. Cuvettes for use in spectrophotometry must be properly matched.

7. Spectrophotometric assays are performed with either a one point calibration or a standard curve.

8. One point calibration assays require that a standard solution be assayed with each patient sample.

9. Standard curves are prepared by measuring the absorbance of serial dilutions of a standard and plotting these against concentration.

10. For a substance to be quantified with a photometric analysis, the test system must follow Beer's law.

11. All veterinary practice laboratories must ensure that employees adhere to written laboratory safety practices.

12. An effective quality control program is essential to ensuring that test results are accurate.

REVIEW QUESTIONS

1. Differentiate between achromatic and planachromatic lens types.
2. Describe the procedure for calibration of the refractometer.
3. Which pipette is the most accurate of the multigraduated pipettes?
4. True or False. Microliter pipettes always require rinsing.
5. True or False. Transfer pipettes are the most accurate single volume pipettes.
6. True or False. A "to deliver" pipette should have the last drop of liquid blown out of the tip of the pipette.
7. Match the following:
   a) milli   1) 0.1
   b) nano   2) 0.01
   c) micro   3) 0.001
   d) deci   4) 0.000001
   e) centi   5) 0.000000001

8. What is the function of the monochromator in the spectrophotometer?
9. Matched cuvettes demonstrate transmission within _____ % of each other.
10. Write the general equation for determining concentration of a substance with a one point calibration.
11. If a standard solution of 80 mg/dl is diluted 1:5, 1:10, and 1:20, what is the final concentration of standard in each of the dilutions?
12. If a test system complies with Beer's law, what is the relationship between concentration, absorbance, and transmission?
13. The government agency which mandates safety in the workplace is the _____ .
14. Define precision and accuracy.
15. List at lease two sources of error in clinical laboratory testing.

ANSWERS TO REVIEW QUESTIONS

1. Planachromatic lenses provide a flat field of view on which the entire field is in focus. Achromatic lenses exhibit some blurriness, especially around the edges of the microscopic field.
2. A few drops of distilled water are placed on the optical surface of the instrument and the hinged cover put in place. The instrument should read 1.00 with distilled water.
3. The Mohr measuring pipette is the most accurate multigraduated pipette.
4. True. Microliter pipettes always require rinsing and should be used only when liquid is already present in the vessel into which you are pipetting.
5. False. Transfer pipettes are not graduated and cannot be used to measure volume. The most accurate single gradation pipettes are volumetric pipettes.
6. False. A "to deliver" pipette is usually, but not always, calibrated as "with blow-out." The pipette will contain a double etched or frosted band if blow-out is required.
7. a) 3   b) 5   c) 4   d) 1   e) 2
8. The monochromator fragments light into equally dispersed segments.
9. Matched cuvettes demonstrate transmission within 1% of each other.
10. $$\text{Concentration of patient sample} = \frac{\text{Abs. of sample} \times \text{Concentration of standard}}{\text{Abs. of standard}}$$
11. The 1:5 dilution contains 16 mg/dl, 1:10 contains 8 mg/dl, and 1:20 contains 4 mg/dl.
12. Concentration is directly related to absorbance in a linear fashion and inversely and logarithmically related to transmission.
13. The Occupational Safety and Health Administration mandates safety in the workplace.
14. Precision refers to the reproducibility of a test result. Accuracy refers to the closeness with which a test result approximates the "true" value.
15. Common sources of error include use of dirty glassware, inappropriate use of pipettes, failure to properly calibrate and maintain instruments, improper sample collection and handling, etc.

SELECTED READING

Carreiro-Lewandowski E, Duben-VonLaufen JL, Bishop JL: *Laboratory Manual for Clinical Chemistry*. Philadelphia, 1987, JB Lippincott.

Kaplan A, Szabo L: *Clinical Chemistry: interpretation and techniques*, ed 2. St. Louis, 1983, CV Mosby Co.

Tietz NW, editor: *Textbook of Clinical Chemistry*, Philadelphia, 1986, WB Saunders Co.

Coles EH: *Veterinary Clinical Pathology*, ed 4. Philadelphia, 1986, WB Saunders Co.

Benjamin M: *Outline of Veterinary Clinical Pathology*, ed 3. Ames, IA, 1978, Iowa State University Press.

Mukherjee KL: *Review of Clinical Laboratory Methods*. St. Louis, 1979, CV Mosby Co.

Bishop ML, Duben-Engelkerk JL, Fody EP: *Clinical Chemistry: principles, procedures & correlations*. Philadelphia, 1992, JB Lippincott.

Clerc JM: *An Introduction to Clinical Laboratory Science*. St. Louis, 1982, CV Mosby Co.

Hematology

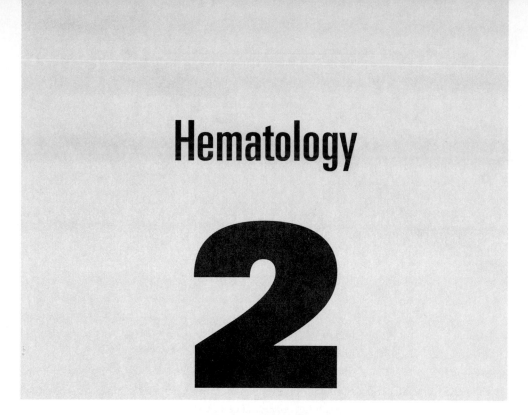

PERFORMANCE OBJECTIVES
After completion of this chapter, the student will:

Describe the procedure for harvesting serum from a blood sample.

List the phases of hematopoiesis and describe the events that occur in each stage.

List the hematopoietic organs and identify the role of each in the hematopoietic process.

List the cells in the erythrocyte maturation process
and identify the general trends seen in cell development.

Describe the synthesis of hemoglobin, the aging
process in the erythrocyte, and subsequent breakdown of hemoglobin.

List the functions of the erythrocyte.

Describe the stages in maturation of granulocytes.

List the functions of each of the blood leukocytes.

Explain how species variations in
neutrophil:lymphocyte ratios are reflected in the species' response to disease.

Describe the steps in the inflammatory response.

Describe the appearance and function of the thrombocytes.

Describe routine blood collection protocols in various species,
including source, site, animal restraint, and equipment selection.

Define "anticoagulant" and explain the
mechanism by which each type of anticoagulant functions.

HEMATOLOGY

Hematology can be defined as the study of blood and the blood-forming organs. In clinical practice, this study is normally limited to evaluation of the cellular components of blood. The noncellular, or plasma portion of the blood accounts for approximately 55% of the total blood volume. It is composed of more than 90% water, 7% protein of various types, and the remainder of other substances, such as vitamins, hormones, etc. The cellular elements comprise 45% of the total blood volume and are of three types: erythrocytes (red blood cells), leukocytes (white blood cells), and thrombocytes (platelets). A basic understanding of the formation, appearance, and function of these cells is essential for their proper evaluation by the laboratory technician. The technician must also ensure that appropriate blood collection procedures have been followed and the samples handled correctly.

HEMATOPOIESIS

Hematopoiesis (production of blood cells) occurs in several phases beginning in early embryonic life.

The *Mesoblastic Phase* of hematopoiesis occurs during the first quarter of embryonic development. Mesenchyme, the embryonic connective tissue, differentiates to form the endothelial lining of the first blood vessels. The more centrally located elements of these vessels become the blood cells. Large nucleated cells which contain hemoglobin are formed.

Erythropoiesis (production of erythrocytes) in the liver, spleen, and thymus marks the beginning of the *Hepatic Phase*. Nucleated red blood cells, granulocytes, and megakaryocytes are formed. Some agranulocytes are also formed.

Bone marrow granulopoiesis begins by the second half of gestation and marks the beginning of the *Myeloid Phase*. Erythropoietic activity in the liver begins to decrease as the bone marrow gradually takes over this function. The primitive mesenchymal cells are reduced to a minimum. These cells retain their pluripotentiality and persist throughout life.

In the young animal, all bones contain red marrow and are hematopoietically active. As the animal matures, much of the red marrow is replaced by yellow marrow, particularly in the long bones. Red marrow, and thus hematopoietic activity, is retained primarily in the flat bones. Some primitive stem cells remain in the long bones. Under conditions of high blood cell demand, the yellow marrow can be reclaimed for hematopoiesis.

Hematopoietic organs

The organs involved in the production of blood serve a variety of functions. They may produce blood cells or components of the cells. They may also act as storage organs for these cells and components. In addition, these organs may perform regulatory functions.

Bone marrow

In the adult animal, the red bone marrow is the primary site for production and maturation of blood cells and platelets. In addition, the bone marrow is a storage area for these cells and for iron.

Liver

The liver is a prominent site of prenatal hematopoiesis. Storage of iron and B vitamins and production of plasma proteins are also hematopoietic functions of the liver.

Kidney

The kidneys perform a regulatory function in the formation of blood and maintenance of homeostasis. The plasma protein concentration and blood pressure are regulated by the kidney. The kidneys are also the major source of the hormone erythropoietin. This hormone targets the bone marrow and is the primary stimulus for erythrocyte production.

Lymph nodes

Lymph node tissue is a site for maturation of lymphocytes and is involved in the production of antibodies.

Spleen

Some prenatal hematopoiesis occurs in the spleen. In the adult, the spleen acts as a reservoir for storage of red blood cells and iron. Agranulocytes are also stored and matured here.

Stomach

Hydrochloric acid in the stomach converts dietary iron to an absorbable form for red blood cell production. The stomach also contains an enzyme necessary for the absorption of vitamin B_{12}.

Thymus

The thymus produces thymic factor, a hormone necessary for the normal development of the thymus-dependent or T-lymphocytes. This gland is largest in late prenatal and early postnatal life and atrophies later in life.

ERYTHROPOIESIS

Cells of the kidneys monitor the balance of oxygen in the tissues. In response to tissue hypoxia, these cells stimulate the production and release of erythropoietin. This hormone travels via the bloodstream to the bone marrow, where it stimulates mitosis of the hemacytoblast, or primitive stem cell. Erythropoietin also stimulates the hemacytoblast to differentiate to a rubriblast. Rubriblasts are highly mitotic and each can give rise to as many as sixteen red blood cells. Further development of the cell continues in the bone marrow through the following stages: (1) prorubricyte, (2) rubricyte, (3) metarubricyte, (4) reticulocyte, (5) erythrocyte. As this maturation progresses, some general trends in cell development are seen. Early in maturation, the cells are large, the cytoplasm stains dark purple or blue, and the nucleus appears dark, coarse, and large. As the cell continues to develop, the nuclear size gradually decreases. The cell becomes smaller and the cytoplasm stains pink. Maturation through the metarubricyte stage must occur in the bone marrow and is usually completed in about 72 hours. If released into peripheral circulation, the metarubricyte will not continue to mature. Reticulocytes are capable of completing development once released from the bone marrow. A description of the immature cells in the erythrocyte maturation series is given in Table 2-1. In many species, both reticulocytes and mature erythrocytes are normally found in circulation.

HEMOGLOBIN SYNTHESIS

The hemoglobin molecule is the functional unit of the erythrocyte. Hemoglobin is a quaternary protein with two main components: heme, which contains iron, and globin, which consists of paired chains of amino acids. Synthesis of hemoglobin begins during the mesoblastic phase of hematopoiesis in early embryonic life and occurs primarily in the rubricytic phase of erythropoiesis. A number of dietary and hormonal factors are necessary for hemoglobin production. Adequate protein intake is of primary importance. Iron and B vitamins are essential parts of the molecule. Cobalt and copper are also utilized in synthesis, although these are not present in the final molecule.

The two sets of polypeptide chains which comprise the globin portion of the molecule are assembled by the ribosome in the cytoplasm of the immature erythrocyte. The specific types of chains will vary according to the stage of pre- and postnatal life. The first chains are designated epsilon (E). In the early embryo, four E chains are incorporated into the molecule. In later fetal life, these are replaced with two delta chains and two alpha chains. Adult hemoglobin consists of 2 alpha and 2 beta chains.

TABLE 2-1
Erythrocyte maturation cell characteristics

Name	Nucleus Size	Nucleus Chromatin	Mitotic activity	Nucleoli	Cytoplasm	Hemoglobin synthesis
Rubriblast	Large	Coarsely stippled	High	Many	Greenish-blue	None
Prorubricyte	Becomes smaller	Dense	Continues	Present, indistinct	Basophilia	None
Rubricyte	Smaller	Clumped	Peaks	None	Basophilia, polychromasia	Peaks
Metarubricyte	Pyknotic, extruded, or fragmented		None	None	Acidophilia,	Tapers off
Reticulocyte	None		None	None	Polychromasia	None
Erythrocyte	None		None	None	Orthochromic	None

Each of the four polypeptide chains has a heme molecule attached which is produced in the bone marrow. Amino acids and enzymes are joined into a pyrrole ring compound and are acted upon enzymatically to form protoporphyrin. One ferrous iron molecule binds to each of the four heme molecules and is located in a loop of each of the polypeptide chains.

ERYTHROCYTE CHARACTERISTICS

The erythrocyte is the most numerous cellular element found in blood and is composed primarily of water (60% to 70%). Another 28% to 35% of the cell is hemoglobin and the remaining 5% consists of organic and inorganic material such as salts and organelles. The red blood cells of most mammalian species are anuclear and appear flat and disc-shaped with little or no central depression. One notable exception to this general description is the canine erythrocyte, which is a biconcave disk with a distinct area of central pallor. Avian and reptilian red blood cells are generally oval with a prominent nucleus.

ERYTHROCYTE FUNCTION

Red blood cells are primarily carriers of hemoglobin and, as such, increase the efficiency of oxygen transport. They also contribute to optimum fluid dynamics of blood and to blood volume by means of their mass. Oxygen binds to hemoglobin in the lungs and is exchanged for carbon dioxide at tissue sites. This process occurs as a result of simple diffusion along a pressure and concentration gradient. Hemoglobin exists in several forms, and the transformation from one form to another results in a conformational change in the molecule which is responsible for the rapid and efficient oxygen/carbon dioxide exchange that occurs.

Energy in the form of ATP is required in order for the cell to maintain the oxygen-binding ability of hemoglobin and to maintain the integrity of the cell membrane and the osmotic and ionic equilibrium. Mature red blood cells lack a nucleus and therefore must rely on a modification of glycolysis for energy. ATP is synthesized by utilizing the enzyme glucose-6-phosphate-dehydrogenase (G-6-PD) to catalyze the oxidation and reduction of hemoglobin.

Once released from the bone marrow, the erythrocyte has a finite life span which is variable among species. As the cell ages, a deficiency of G-6-PD develops which leads to the production of abnormal hemoglobin. This abnormal hemoglobin alters the cell membrane and triggers the removal of the cell by macrophages in the spleen.

FORMS OF HEMOGLOBIN

Oxygen bound to hemoglobin forms the compound oxyhemoglobin. This process reverses when oxygen is released at tissue sites and diffuses into cells. Carbon dioxide then diffuses into the erythrocyte.

Free hemoglobin in the plasma may be oxidized to methemoglobin, in which the iron is in the ferric ($+3$) state. This form is relatively inefficient at oxygen transport but can be reduced during RBC metabolism. The enzyme methemoglobin reductase (MR) facilitates this reaction and prevents buildup of this form in the blood. Genetic enzyme deficiency or certain oxidant drugs can cause increased levels of methemoglobin and manifest as a bluish discoloration of mucous membranes.

Carboxyhemoglobin results from exposure to carbon monoxide, which binds hemoglobin with an affinity 210 times greater than oxygen and is therefore essentially irreversible. Exposure to carbon monoxide gives a cherry red color to blood and mucous membranes.

Sulfhemoglobin can be derived from either hemoglobin or methemoglobin reacting with hydrogen sulfide. This occurs as a result of normal RBC aging processes or drug toxicity. This reaction is irreversible, and this form cannot bind oxygen.

Exposure to certain types of cyanide will convert all forms of hemoglobin, except sulfhemoglobin, to cyanmethemoglobin. This reaction is the basis for the most commonly performed hemoglobin assay, since it provides the capability to measure nearly all populations of hemoglobin in the blood.

LEUKOPOIESIS

The stimulus for development of white blood cells is believed to be under hormonal influence. As with erythropoiesis, leukopoiesis begins with stimulation of the stem cell. The pattern of development varies depending on the ultimate fate of the cell. As with erythrocyte maturation, some general trends are seen as leukocytes develop. The earlier stages are large cells with a large nuclear to cytoplasm ratio. Nucleoli are present and cytoplasm is basophilic. As these cells mature, size gradually decreases, nucleoli become less prominent, and specific cytoplasmic granules may appear.

White blood cells are divided into two categories depending on the presence or absence of cytoplasmic granules. Granulocytes are further divided and named according to the staining pattern of their cytoplasm and granules on a routine Wright's stained blood film. The cells within the granulocytic series are the neutrophils, eosinophils, and basophils. The agranulocytic cell types are the lymphocytes and monocytes.

Granulocytes

Neutrophils, eosinophils, and basophils show similar maturation patterns. The stages in the maturation of granulocytes are: (1) myeloblast, (2) promyelocyte, (3) myelocyte, (4) metamyelocyte, (5) band, (6) segmented. The myeloblast is similar morphologically and therefore difficult to distinguish from the lymphocytic blast cell. Mitotic activity is high and continues into the promyelocyte stage. The production of specific granules begins during the myelocyte stage, and these cells are the most actively mitotic. Mitotic activity ceases by the metamyelocyte stage. The nucleus of the metamyelocyte is greatly condensed. In some species, particularly birds, reptiles, and pigs, these cells may normally be found in circulation.

Agranulocytes

The mature monocyte seen in circulation is not a fully developed cell. Monocytes represent one stage in the development of the tissue macrophage. The formation of monocytes originates with stem cells that differentiate to monoblasts. An intermediate form, the promonocyte, can also be identified in the bone marrow.

Lymphocytes have a complex pattern of development and maturation. The cell line orginates from the same bone marrow stem cells that are capable of producing all the blood cells. Two immature stages, the lymphoblast and prolymphocyte, can be identified. Maturation may occur in the bone marrow or in the lymphoid organs, particularly the thymus. Lymphocytes that are derived from the bone marrow are designated B lymphocytes. Those that are matured in the thymus are designated T lymphocytes. T and B lymphocytes can not be differentiated by using ordinary staining techniques. These two subpopulations have diverse functions which will be discussed in Chapter 5.

LEUKOCYTE CHARACTERISTICS

Granulocytes

Neutrophils are the most numerous white blood cells found in most mammalian species. The nucleus is segmented into 3 to 5 lobes. In most species, thin filaments can be seen which connect the lobes. These filaments are not present between the lobes of canine neutrophils and are rarely seen in feline neutrophils. The nucleus stains deep reddish-purple and the chromatin has a coarse, clumped texture. Cytoplasm is abundant, usually stains pale pink, and contains numerous fine granules which stain pinkish-lilac.

Eosinophils are usually the largest of the granulocytes in normal mammalian blood. The nucleus is segmented into two large lobes and the chromatin is coarse and clumped. Cytoplasm is abundant and is usually colorless to light blue. Eosinophilic granules vary in size and number depending on the species being examined, but they are generally large and somewhat refractile. In the feline, the granules are often rod shaped. Canine granules vary in size and are smaller in number. The equine has large distinct granules that stain bright orange. In the bovine, these granules are small, round, and uniform in size and often completely fill the cytoplasm.

Basophils also have a segmented nucleus, but the lobes are difficult to discern as they tend to crowd together and are often obscured by cytoplasmic granules. The chromatin material is less coarse than in the other granulocytes. Cytoplasm is light pink to colorless and usually contains prominent irregular granules which stain purplish-black. The feline basophil has fewer distinct granules than most mammalian species. If the blood smear is overwashed, granules may be removed and the cell confused with a vacuolated monocyte.

Agranulocytes

The largest of the cells in peripheral circulation are the monocytes, which range from 14μ to 20μ in diameter. The nucleus may be round, bean shaped, indented, or folded and has a soft, spongy appearance which stains pale bluish-violet. Chromatin material is fine and skein-like. Cytoplasm is abundant, appears opaque, and stains blue-gray. Fine lilac granules may be seen and give the cytoplasm a "ground glass" appearance. Vacuoles are frequently present and blunt pseudopods may be seen.

Lymphocytes vary markedly in size from 7μ to 18μ, depending on the origin and function of the cell. These size variations are primarily due to different amounts of cytoplasm. The lymphocytic nucleus is slightly larger than a normal red blood cell and is usually round or oval in shape. A slightly indented nucleus may be found in the normal bovine. Chromatin material is very dense and clumped, especially in small lymphocytes. Cytoplasm amounts vary from a very thin ring of blue cytoplasm around the nucleus of a small lymphocyte to abundant, pale blue, transparent cytoplasm of larger lymphocytes. Granules are not usually present, but a few large lysosomes can occasionally be seen.

LEUKOCYTE FUNCTION

In addition to those leukocytes in circulation, a large number of leukocytes are found in the marginal pool. The marginal pool refers to those leukocytes which are physically located along the blood vessel walls and are not freely circulating in the plasma. These cells may represent as much as two to three times the abundance of the circulating leukocytes. With the exception of the lymphocyte, the principle function of leukocytes is phagocytosis and they function almost exclusively within tissue spaces. Neutrophils are involved in phagocytosis of microorganisms and other foreign particles and in the initiation of an inflammatory response. Basophils also assist in the initiation of an inflammatory response by the release of histamine, heparin, and serotonin from their granules. The eosinophil is involved in the control of the inflammatory reaction. This control is initiated by the release of the eosinophilic granules which contain agents to deactivate histamine and heparin and thus have an antiinflammatory effect.

Monocytes are also phagocytic cells and are responsible for the removal of dead cells, cell fragments, microorganisms, and insoluble particles from both the blood and body tissues. Lymphocytes are primarily involved in the immune response and in the production of antibody.

LEUKOCYTE LIFE SPAN

White blood cells are matured in the bone marrow and released into the bloodstream. Most remain in circulation for only a few hours before entering the tissues. Once in a tissue space, granulocytes and monocytes are unable to return to peripheral circulation. In general, the shorter their life span in circulation, the greater the likelihood of finding immature forms in the peripheral blood. The "T lymphocyte" is the longest lived of all leukocytes. Its life span is thought to be up to 20 years and it is capable of traveling between blood and tissue spaces and back again as needed.

LEUKOCYTE RESPONSE

Any type of acute insult to the organism will result in the release of hormones which prevent the margination of neutrophils. The degree of neutrophilia (increase in neutrophil numbers) exhibits species variability. This variability is reflected in the neutrophil to lymphocyte ratio of a particular species (Table 2-2). The canine has a relatively large N:L ratio of 3.5. As a result, the dog will show a neutrophilia very early on in the course of a disease process. In the bovine, the N:L ratio is relatively small, about 0.5. A pathologic condition is usually greatly advanced before a neutropenia is evident.

The neutrophil also has the initiating role in the inflammatory response. In response to chemotactic factors released by damaged cells, neutrophils marginate and enter tissue spaces. Neutrophilic granules contain lysozymes which aid phagocytosis of an infectious agent or dead and damaged tissue. Basophils also enter the site and the release of their heparin-containing granules helps keep capillaries free of clots. Basophils also release histamine granules which helps keep blood vessels dilated. Eosinophils release granules which counteract the action of histamine and are an important factor in control of inflammation. As this process progresses, the pH begins to drop in the area and the neutrophils become unable to function. Monocytes will then enter the area and pick up the phagocytic activity.

THROMBOCYTES

Thrombocytes, or platelets, are cytoplasmic fragments of the bone marrow megakaryocyte. They vary in size from 1 to 4 μm and may have multiple pointed projections. They are generally round, oval, or spindle-shaped and stain pale blue with purplish granules.

THROMBOCYTE FUNCTION

Platelets contribute to hemostasis by providing an initiating coagulation factor (platelet factor III) and by mechanically plugging small breaks in small blood vessels. This aspect will be discussed further in Chapter 4.

TABLE 2-2
N:L ratios

Species	N:L ratio
Canine	3.5
Feline	1.8
Equine	1.1
Bovine	0.5

BLOOD SAMPLE RECORD

Date _2/8/94_

Patient Name _Bijou_

Owner Name _King_

Species _K9_   Sex _♀_   Age _6½ y_

~~Preprandial~~ or Postprandial?

Type of sample(s) _whole blood (venous)_

Anticoagulant(s) _EDTA_

Treatment(s) given prior to sampling ____

_NA_

Comments: _____

_____

Test(s) Requested _CBC w/ diff_

_____

_____

Fig. 2-1. Example of completed blood sample record.

COLLECTION AND HANDLING OF BLOOD

A number of factors must be considering before performing blood collection. Improper blood collection procedures may make samples unsuitable for analysis. Specific blood collection protocols vary depending on the patient species, the volume of blood needed, the method of restraint, and the type of sample needed. A blood collection record should be maintained for each sample (Fig. 2-1). The record should include a brief patient medical history and any remarks regarding the actual collection procedure (i.e., chemical restraint used, patient upset, etc.). All patients should be fasted for 6 to 12 hours before scheduled blood collection. If the animal has eaten recently, this must also be noted on the blood sample record.

Blood source

Venous blood is usually preferred and is suitable for all testing except pH and blood gas measurements. In most species, veins are easily accessible and good volume can be obtained with minimal trauma. Most normal value charts provide reference values for venous blood.

Arterial blood samples are sometimes required when measurements of blood gases or pH are requested. These are more difficult to obtain and the procedure is often painful to the animal.

Capillary or peripheral blood is collected from a superficial wound in a capillary bed, typically the nail bed. This type of sample may be used when small volumes and repeated testing is needed.

Site selection

Blood collection sites are usually dependent on the size of the animal and the volume of blood needed (Table 2-3). For most dogs and some cats, the cephalic vein is preferred. In small dogs or cats, this vessel can be used provided a large volume of blood is not needed. The saphenous vein may also be used but is more difficult to stabilize. For large volumes, jugular veinipuncture is recommended. Although slightly more traumatic, this method can yield a large amount of blood. The jugular vein is also the preferred site for blood collection in horses and is often used in cows.

For avian patients, the wing vein may be used if a large volume is needed. For smaller volumes, a nail can be clipped and the blood collected into a capillary tube.

Cardiac puncture and intraorbital sinus bleeding can be performed in small laboratory or exotic animals. Both of these methods require that the animal be anesthetized.

TABLE 2-3
Commonly used blood collection sites

Canine	Cephalic vein
	Jugular vein
	Saphenous vein
Feline	Cephalic vein
	Jugular vein
Equine	Jugular vein
Bovine	Caudal vein
	Mammary vein
	Jugular vein
Avian	Wing vein
	Toenail clip
Rabbit	Ear vein
	Toenail clip
Rodents	Tail vein
	Cardiac puncture

Site preparation

The site should be clipped of hair and scrubbed with alcohol. The alcohol should be allowed to evaporate before beginning the procedure. Excess alcohol must be avoided as it increases the likelihood of sample hemolysis.

Restraint

Restraint of the animal during blood collection is usually required. Minimal manual restraint is preferred whenever possible. Mechanical restraining devices can be used, but these often upset the animal. This stress can lead to splenic contraction which will alter the hematologic parameters. Chemical restraint is sometimes needed for particularly fractious animals. If used, this should always be noted on the blood collection record as some pharmocologic agents will interfere with certain test methodologies.

Collection equipment

The type of blood collection equipment used will depend on the source of the blood. For arterial blood samples, a needle and glass syringe are required and the sample requires special handling. Air must be expelled from the syringe before use and the tip immediately sealed following sample collection.

Venous blood samples can be collected using either a glass or plastic syringe or a vacuum system. If a syringe/needle system is chosen, plastic syringes are preferred since platelets can aggregate on the inner walls of glass syringes and thus interefere with thrombocyte measurements. Needle size is chosen based on the size of the animal. In general, the largest bore size possible should be used. For most small animals, 20 to 22 gauge needles are appropriate. The use of smaller needles can result in trauma to the blood cells and hemolysis of the sample. The needle must be removed from the syringe before transferring the blood into a tube. Erythrocytes may rupture (hemolyze) if forced back through the needle.

The vacuum system is ideal when multiple samples are needed. A single veinipuncture can yield samples which are adequate for all types of testing. An evacuated tube, disposable needle, and needle holder are utilized and blood is collected directly into glass tubes which may be plain or contain a premeasured amount of anticoagulant. A fixed amount of blood is drawn into the tube based on the strength of the vacuum. The tube is then withdrawn from the needle and additional tubes can be inserted. It is important that the proper size tube be used as a tube that is too large can collapse the vein.

Peripheral blood is usually collected directly into a capillary tube. A sterile lancet may be used to make a superficial wound in a capillary bed. The most common method for collection of peripheral blood is a toenail clip. The wound must not be squeezed as this will contaminate the sample with tissue fluid. The first few drops will also be contaminated with fluid and cellular debris and must be wiped away before the sample collection begins.

Anticoagulants

An anticoagulant is a chemical which interferes with the blood clotting mechanisms, either permanently or temporarily. The technician must ensure that the anticoagulant chosen does not interfere with the blood constituent being assayed (Table 2-4).

Evaluations which require whole blood samples must be immediately mixed with an appropriate anticoagulant. The anticoagulant chosen should be one which preserves the integrity of the cellular components. Isotonic solutions are those which contain the same concentration of dissolved materials as the cells which are suspended in the solution. Solutions that have greater concentrations than the cells are said to be hypertonic. Normal osmotic processes will cause water to be drawn from the cells in an attempt to equilibrate the concentrations in these two areas. This will result in shrinkage of the cells. Similarly, hypotonic solutions which have a lesser concentration of solute material than the cells will result in swelling of the cell as water from the surrounding fluid is drawn into the cells. The anticoagulant chosen must be isotonic for blood cells.

The most commonly used anticoagulant for hematology studies is a sodium or potassium salt of ethylenediaminetetraacetic acid (EDTA). EDTA effectively removes calcium from the clot reaction, is irreversible and toxic. It is available in either a liquid or powder form. The liquid form should be avoided as it dilutes the sample. Excess EDTA shrinks cells. The amount of EDTA used must be in proportion to the sample size.

Citrate and oxalate anticoagulants are used primarily for coagulation studies when plasma samples are required. Both have temporary, reversible effects on the clotting mechanisms. They are available as sodium, potassium, ammonium, or lithium salts. These salts will interfere with some biochemical testing and will damage erythrocytes. They are generally not suitable for hematology because they may shrink cells. Citrates are nontoxic and are often used for blood transfusions. Oxalates are toxic and hypertonic to red blood cells.

TABLE 2-4
Commonly used anticoagulants

Name	Mode of action	Advantages	Disadvantages	Uses
Heparin	Antithrombin	Reversible, nontoxic	Clumps WBCs, expensive	Critical RBC measurements
EDTA (K^+, Na^+)	Chelates Ca^+	Best preservation	Irreversible, shrinks cells	Hematology
Oxalates (K^+, Na^+, Li^+)	Chelates Ca^+	Temporary	Variable effects	Coagulation
Citrates (Na^+, Li^+)	Chelates Ca^+	Nontoxic, reversible	Interferes with blood chemistry	Coagulation transfusions
Flourides (Na^+)	Chelates Ca^+	Inhibits cell metabolism	Interferes with enzymatic tests	Preserves blood glucose

Heparin anticoagulants are useful where critical red blood cell measurements are needed and may be used for plasma collection. Heparin is unsuitable for white blood cell analyses as it may cause the cells to clump and it interferes with their normal staining patterns.

Fluoride inhibits in vitro glycolysis by blood cells and is a useful anticoagulant when preservation of glucose is critical.

SPECIMEN HANDLING

All specimen tubes must be labeled with the patient and owner's name, the date the sample was drawn, and the type of anticoagulant, if any.

For whole blood samples, blood is drawn into a tube with the proper amount and type of anticoagulant. The tube is then mixed by gentle inversion. Metabolism of blood cells continues after the blood is removed from the patient. Refrigeration will slow the metabolic rate and any specimen that is not to be used immediately must be refrigerated and then remixed before testing. Samples that are held for an excessive amount of time before testing (more than one hour at room temperature) will often show variation in the cells. Any delays in performing hematology tests must be noted along with the results of the tests. Plasma samples are obtained by mixing the blood with an appropriate anticoagulant and then centrifuging for 10 to 20 minutes at 1000 G. A Pasteur pipette is used to remove the plasma to a separate container. The plasma may be refrigerated or frozen. Stored plasma samples may develop fibrin clots and would require recentrifugation before testing.

Serum samples are obtained by drawing the blood into a plain sterile or serum separator tube. The sample should be left undisturbed at room temperature for 20 to 30 minutes while the clot is forming. After clotting, a wooden applicator is used to gently separate the clot from the wall of the tube. The tube is then centrifuged for 10 to 20 minutes at 1000 G. The serum is removed with a Pasteur pipette and refrigerated or frozen if testing is delayed. Numerous blood constituents may be altered if cells are allowed to remain in contact with serum or plasma.

AMOUNT OF BLOOD REQUIRED

In general, a blood sample will yield approximately half of its volume in serum or plasma. In patients that are dehydrated, this yield will be reduced in proportion to the percent dehydration. The minimum amount of serum or plasma needed varies depending on the types of testing. The technician should be familiar with the volumes used for each of the tests desired. The amount taken should be at least double the minimum needed. This will allow adequate volume should repeat testing be needed due to errors or equipment malfunction. Repeat testing may also be required if a measurement exceeds the equipment capabilities. In this case, the sample would be diluted and reexamined.

Bone marrow sampling

Bone marrow samples may be collected from the humerus, at the crest of the ilium, femur, or sternum of the dog. The femur is the preferred site for marrow collection in the cat. In the bovine and equine, the rib or sternum is preferred. The sample is collected utilizing a bone marrow aspiration needle with a syringe attached. All equipment must be sterile and the skin over the collection site clipped free of hair and disinfected. Aseptic surgical technique must be used to avoid marrow infection. Smears for differential cell examination should be made from the few drops of marrow on the tip of the needle immediately following collection. The remainder of the sample may be mixed with EDTA. Granular marrow material is sometimes preserved in a fixative, such as formalin, for later analysis.

The bone marrow smear must be carefully made to avoid artifact due to excess pressure. Distortion of the cells must be avoided. A fine brush is sometimes utilized for preparation of the bone marrow smear. Excess blood is removed by touching a capillary tube to the slide and allowing the blood to fill the tube. Bone marrow granules may also be used to prepare a 'squash' preparation. Staining of the smear is often accomplished with a Wright's stain, or a vital stain may sometimes be used.

KEY POINTS

1. The hormone erythropoietin is released in response to tissue hypoxia and stimulates erythropoiesis.

2. Maturation of erythrocytes occurs in the bone marrow.

3. Hemoglobin is a quaternary protein which contains two pairs of polypeptide chains.

4. Erythrocytes are carriers of hemoglobin and therefore function in oxygen and carbon dioxide transport.

5. Erythrocyte metabolism consists of a modification of glycolysis which requires the enzyme G-6-PD.

6. Any condition which is characterized by abnormal hemoglobin will cause a distortion in the erythrocyte membrane and shorten the cell's life span.

7. Hemoglobin can exist in several forms. Some of these forms are not efficient at oxygen transport and can be harmful.

8. The blood leukocytes are classified based on the presence or absence of specific cytoplasmic granules.

9. The primary function of granulocytes and monocytes is phagocytosis.

10. Lymphocytes are components of the immune system.

11. The degree of species variability in response to disease is reflected in the neutrophil:lymphocyte ratio.

12. Blood collection protocols vary depending on the size of the animal, the volume of blood needed, and the type of sample needed.

13. A blood collection record should be completed for each patient and accompany the sample to the lab.

14. Anticoagulants are chemicals that inhibit or prevent clotting, either permanently or temporarily.

15. The volume of blood collected should be at least double the minimum needed.

16. Thrombocytes are cytoplasmic fragments of the bone marrow megakaryocyte that function in blood coagulation.

REVIEW QUESTIONS

1. List the cells in the erythrocyte maturation series.
2. The greatest amount of hemoglobin is produced during the _____ phase of erythropoiesis.
3. What is the function of G-6-PD in the erythrocyte?
4. What is the role of methemoglobin reductase in the erythrocyte?
5. What is the role of the monocyte in the inflammatory response?
6. What type of polypeptide chains are present in adult hemoglobin?
7. The _____ vein is recommended for blood collection in most animals.
8. Why should the alcohol used to clean the blood collection site be allowed to dry before proceeding with blood collection?
9. The use of small gauge needles for blood collection could cause _____ of erythrocytes.
10. The anticoagulant of choice for most hematologic testing is _____.
11. The most commonly used anticoagulants for coagulation testing are _____.
12. _____ anticoagulants provide the best preservation of glucose.
13. A blood sample will yield approximately _____ its volume in serum or plasma.

ANSWERS TO REVIEW QUESTIONS

1. The cells in the erythrocyte maturation series are: (1) prorubricyte, (2) rubricyte, (3) metarubricyte, (4) reticulocyte, and (4) erythrocyte.
2. The greatest amount of hemoglobin is synthesized during the rubricytic phase of erythropoiesis.
3. In the erythrocyte, G-6-PD is used during ATP synthesis to catalyze the oxidation and reduction of hemoglobin.
4. Methemoglobin reductase facilitates the reduction of methemoglobin to free hemoglobin.
5. Monocytes pick up phagocytic activity as inflammation becomes chronic.
6. Adult hemoglobin contains two alpha and two beta polypeptide chains.
7. The jugular vein can be used for blood collection in most animals.
8. To avoid lysis of red blood cells, the alcohol used to clean the blood collection site should be allowed to dry before proceeding.
9. The use of small gauge needles for blood collection could cause lysis or rupture of erythrocytes.
10. The anticoagulant of choice for most hemotologic testing is a sodium or potassium salt of EDTA.
11. The most commonly used anticoagulants for coagulation testing are citrates and oxalates.
12. Fluoride anticoagulants provide the best preservation of glucose.
13. A blood sample will yield approximately half its volume in serum or plasma.

SELECTED READING

Powers LW: *Diagnostic Hematology: clinical and technical principles*. St. Louis, 1989, CV Mosby Co.

Schalm OW, Jain NC, and Carroll EJ: *Veterinary Hematology*, ed 3. Philadelphia, 1975, Lea & Febiger.

Bunn HF, Forget BG: *Hemoglobin: molecular, genetic, and clinical aspects*. Philadelphia, 1986, WB Saunders.

Lewis HB, Rebar AH: *Bone Marrow Evaluation in Veterinary Practice*. St. Louis, 1979, Ralston Purina Co.

Coles EH: *Veterinary Clinical Pathology*, ed 4. Philadelphia, 1986, WB Saunders.

Benjamin M: *Outline of Veterinary Clinical Pathology*, ed 3. Ames, IA, 1978, Iowa State University Press.

Doxey DL: *Clinical Pathology and Diagnostic Procedures*, ed 2, London, 1983, Balliere-Tindall.

Jain NC: *Veterinary Hematology*. The Veterinary Clinics of North America, Small Animal Practice, vol 11. Philadelphia, 1981, WB Saunders Co.

The complete blood count

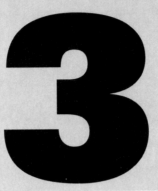

PERFORMANCE OBJECTIVES
After completion of this chapter, the student will:

List the equipment required for manual counting of blood cells.

Explain the general procedure for manual
counting of erythrocytes, leukocytes, and thrombocytes.

Write the general equation for calculation of manual cell counts.

Define the terms "polycythemia" and
"anemia" and list the common causes of these conditions.

Describe the procedure for determining the packed cell volume.

Describe the procedure for determination of the erythrocyte sedimentation rate.

Explain the principle for the
cyanmethemoglobin procedure for hemoglobin determination.

Describe the procedure for determination of erythrocyte indices.

Describe the procedure for performing a differential blood cell count.

Identify the various types of stains available for blood smears.

Identify the morphologic abnormalities of erythrocytes and leukocytes.

Describe the procedure for indirect measurement of thrombocyte numbers.

Describe the procedure for enumeration of reticulocytes.

Describe the principle and general procedure for erythrocyte osmotic fragility testing.

T he complete blood count includes red and white blood cell counts, a differential blood smear, a packed cell volume (PCV), and hemoglobin measurement. Depending on the type of laboratory, this may be done either manually or with automated equipment.

Counting of erythtocytes and leukocytes

Routine evaluation of blood includes enumeration of the cellular elements as part of the complete blood count. Cell counts require a properly collected and anticoagulated blood sample that is fresh and well-mixed. If the sample has been refrigerated, it must be warmed to room temperature and remixed before use. The blood is then diluted using either glass blood dilution pipettes or the Unopette system.

Blood dilution pipettes consist of a stem portion which is calibrated to provide specific dilution ratios and a bulb or mixing chamber which contains a small bead to facilitate thorough mixing (Fig. 3-1). A rubber aspirating tube with a plastic mouthpiece is attached to the end of the pipette and blood is drawn to the desired calibration mark using gentle suction. Diluent is then drawn up to the upper mark. To minimize measurement error from air bubbles and ensure proper mixing of blood and diluent, it is advisable to roll the pipette slightly between the fingers while filling.

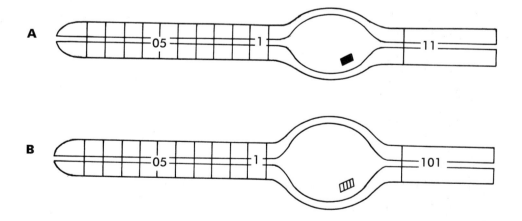

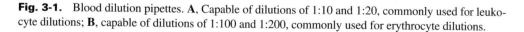

Fig. 3-1. Blood dilution pipettes. **A**, Capable of dilutions of 1:10 and 1:20, commonly used for leukocyte dilutions; **B**, capable of dilutions of 1:100 and 1:200, commonly used for erythrocyte dilutions.

The dilution pipette commonly used for red blood cell counts contains calibrations designated as 0.5, 1, and 101. Since a portion of the diluent remains in the pipette stem and is not mixed with the blood, a total of 100 'parts' of blood plus diluent combines in the bulb. Therefore, filling the pipette with blood to the 1 mark and diluent to the 101 mark results in a dilution ratio of 1:100. Most red cell counts are performed with a dilution ratio of 1:200, which can be achieved by drawing blood to the 0.5 mark and adding diluent. For white blood cell counts, a smaller pipette is normally used which has calibrated marks at 0.5, 1, and 11. Therefore, filling the WBC pipette to the 0.5 mark provides the commonly used dilution ratio of 1:20.

The diluent chosen may vary depending on the laboratory. Diluent for white blood cell counts contains a dilute acid to lyse the red blood cells. Glacial acetic acid is commonly used for white blood cell counts and may have stain added to facilitate visualization of nucleated cells. The red blood cell diluent must be isotonic to maintain the integrity of those more fragile cells. Hayem's dilution fluid and isotonic salt solution are satisfactory dilution fluids for red blood cell counts.

Once properly filled, a rubber pipette closure is applied and the pipette is placed on a pipette shaker for 3 minutes or mixed by hand. If mixing by hand, avoid shaking the pipette on a longitudinal axis as this may force cells into the stem of the pipette and result in dilution error. The diluent in the stem is then discarded and the hemacytometer, or counting chamber, is charged.

The hemacytometer contains two raised bridges which hold the coverglass and two sample counting areas that are completely surrounded by a moat. The coverglass is of optical quality and should never be used for other purposes. The sample counting areas contain a ruled grid, most commonly the Neubauer ruling (Fig. 3-2). The coverglass is applied to the hemacytometer and is then charged with the diluted blood sample. To charge the hemacytometer, simply touch the tip of the pipette to the groove at the lower edge of the coverglass. The sample will flow directly into the ruled area. Care must be taken that the counting area is completely filled and not allowed to overflow into the moat. Should this occur, the hemacytometer should be cleaned and recharged before proceeding. For WBC counts, the hemacytometer should be allowed to sit for up to several minutes in a moist chamber. This will allow the cells to settle while preventing dessication.

The Unopette system is a self-contained semiautomatic blood dilution system which consists of a reservoir and a disposable pipette (Fig. 3-3). The pipettes are available in several sizes and the reservoirs contain a premeasured volume of diluent. To use this system, puncture the diaphragm of the reservoir with the pipette shield. Remove the shield from the reservoir and twist the shield to remove the pipette. Hold the pipette almost horizontally and insert the tip of the pipette into the blood. The pipette will fill by capillary action. Do not remove the pipette from the blood until it is completely filled. Wipe the outside of the pipette to remove the excess blood. Insert the filled pipette into the reservoir while exerting slight pressure by squeezing the reservoir. Releasing the pressure then draws the sample into the diluent. Squeeze the reservoir gently two or three times to rinse the pipette. Be

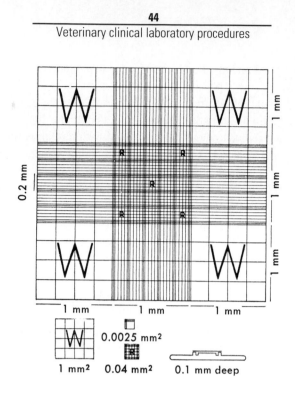

1 mm   1 mm   1 mm

W   0.0025 mm²

1 mm²   0.04 mm²   0.1 mm deep

Fig. 3-2. Hemocytometer grid. Areas marked 'W' are used for leukocyte counts. Areas marked 'R' are used for erythrocyte counts. (Powers LW: *Diagnostic Hematology* 1989, St. Louis, Mosby.)

careful not to expel any liquid through the top of the pipette. Mix by gentle inversion and convert the pipette to a dropper assembly by removing it from the reservoir and replacing it in reverse position. Invert and gently squeeze the reservoir. Discard the first few drops and charge the hemocytometer. White blood cell counts done with the Unopette system generally utilize a 20 μl pipette, which provides a dilution ratio of 1:100. Red blood cell counts are usually performed with 10 μl of sample, for a dilution ratio of 1:200.

Making the count

The Neubauer ruling consists of nine large squares, each measuring 1 mm². The depth of the chamber (distance between the grid area and coverglass) is 0.1 mm. The squares are further subdivided into smaller squares, with the center square, or "super square," being divided into 400 small squares arranged as 25 groups of 16 each.

For dilutions of 1:100, all nine large squares of the grid are counted on each side. Red blood cell counts with a dilution of 1:200 require that the center square and four corner squares of the "super square" be counted. These are general guidelines only, as a specific patient condition, such as severe anemia, may require a different dilution ratio. If more dilute samples are used, more squares should be counted to ensure accuracy.

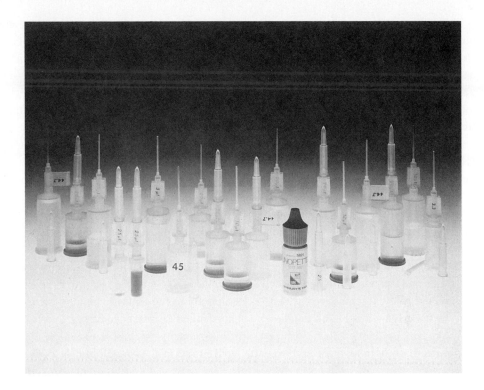

Fig. 3-3. Unopette blood dilution system. (Photo courtesy of Becton-Dickinson VACUTAINER Systems.)

The count should proceed in an orderly fashion, starting at one end of the square, going across to the other side, then down one microscopic field and back across until all cells within the square are counted. Cells that are touching the line between two squares are counted with that square if they are touching either the top or the left line. Do not count cells touching either the bottom or right lines.

The desired squares from each side of the hemacytometer are counted separately and the two numbers are averaged. The number of cells in a microliter of blood is then determined by the following calculation:

$$\frac{\text{\# of cells counted (average of the two sides)}}{\text{(dilution ratio)} \times \text{(volume of one square)} \times \text{(No. of squares counted)}}$$

For example, a red blood cell dilution of 1:200 with five squares in the super square counted on each side of the hemocytometer produced counts of 440 and 460 cells per side; thus

$$\frac{450 \text{ cells}}{1/200 \times 1/10\mu l \times 1/5} = 4,500,000 \text{ cells}/\mu l$$

This value must then be converted to scientific notation. Erythrocyte counts are expressed as the number of cells $\times$ $10^6/\mu l$ and leukocyte counts as the number of cells $\times$ $10^3/\mu l$. Some references may refer to the number of cells per cubic millimeter. One mm^3 is equal to one microliter. For the example above, the value would be $4.5 \times 10^6/\mu l$.

Normal values for erythrocytes should be used as a general guideline only, as this value can be affected by numerous nonpathologic conditions, such as age of the animal, altitude, and body position.

An increase in the circulating red cell mass is termed polycythemia. An apparent polycythemia may be seen in patients with low plasma volume (dehydration). A true polycythemia may result from physiologic rather than pathologic conditions. Newborn mammals may have at least a transient polycythemia. High altitudes will also result in increased red cell mass. More commonly, patients that are stressed by blood collection show a physiologic polycythemia as a result of splenic contraction with subsequent release of red blood cells.

Pathologic polycythemia may be secondary to any condition which causes chronic tissue hypoxia and thus results in bone marrow hyperplasia. The greatest increase in cell numbers is seen in polycythemia vera, which is due directly to hyperplastic bone marrow with no known underlying cause. This condition can appear and disappear suddenly.

Anemia is a reduction in the oxygen-carrying capacity of the blood which may be due to a decrease in number of erythrocytes, concentration of hemoglobin, or both. It is most often secondary to some other disease process, such as blood loss, and may be seen in any condition which causes accelerated destruction or decreased production of red blood cells.

Loss of one third of the total blood volume in 24 hours is termed "acute blood loss." The total red cell count will be reduced and show an increase in reticulocytes and nucleated red blood cells as the bone marrow tries to keep up with the demand. Chronic blood loss frequently involves gastrointestinal bleeding, such as seen with hookworm infections. It may also occur as a result of a coagulation abnormality.

Hemolytic anemias result from increased destruction of red blood cells. This may also be of an acute nature and involve the immune system. Chronic conditions which cause increased intravascular hemolysis include renal disease and splenic dysfunction. Accumulations of urea on the red cell membrane causes distortion of the cell and triggers its early removal from circulation.

A number of conditions can cause a decrease in red cell production. These include ingestion of toxic plants material, such as bracken fern, or chemotherapeutic agents, such as chloramphenicol, which depress the bone marrow erythropoiesis. Nutritional deficiencies and abnormalities in erythropoietin can also result in anemia.

Several classification schemes have been used which categorize anemias according to either morphology or etiology. Morphologic classifications are generally done on the basis of erythrocyte indices (see p. 50).

PACKED CELL VOLUME

The PCV (packed cell volume) is the ratio of red blood cells to total plasma volume and is expressed as a percentage of total blood volume. The procedure can be performed in two ways.

Microhematocrit method

Anticoagulated blood is placed in a plain capillary tube and one end of the tube is sealed with clay. If anticoagulated blood is not available, heparinized capillary tubes may be used. The filled tube is placed in a microhematocrit centrifuge and centrifuged for 5 minutes at 10,000 RPMs. The centrifugal force will layer the blood components according to weight. The heaviest components are the red blood cells and these will be pushed to the bottom of the tube. Above that, a small grayish area designated the "buffy coat" is found (Fig. 3-4). This area consists of white blood cells and thrombocytes. The height of the buffy coat can be used as a rough estimate of total white blood cell count. The presence of increased numbers of nucleated red blood cells in circulation will result in a red tinged buffy coat.

The microhematocrit packed cell volume can be determined using a variety of devices, such as lined cards, wheels, or a ruler. Regardless of the device used, the total height of the column (cells + plasma) and the height of the packed red cell column are measured.

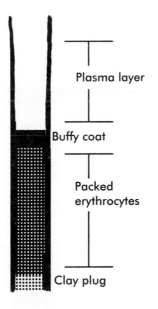

Fig. 3-4. Layers in microhematocrit tube following centrifugation.

Macrohematocrit method

This method is generally more accurate than the microhematocrit method since a larger volume of blood is used. However, in many patients, it may be difficult to obtain an adequate volume of blood to use this method. In addition, this test requires a centrifuge which is capable of maintaining speeds which are beyond the capability of most small, in-house centrifuges. To perform the test, fresh anticoagulated blood is transferred to a Wintrobe tube using a disposable pipette. The pipette should touch the bottom of the tube and be slowly withdrawn as the blood is being expelled. Keep the pipette tip just below the surface of the blood to avoid air bubbles. Fill the Wintrobe tube exactly to the 10 mark. Centrifuge the tube for 10 minutes at 18,000 RPMs and record the level of packed cells by utilizing the scale on the right hand side of the tube. The macrohematocrit ratio is calculated by dividing the level of the packed cells by 10 (the volume of blood in the tube) and multiplying by 100.

Plasma color

Regardless of the method used to determine the packed cell volume, the plasma column should be examined and its color and turbidity evaluated. Normal plasma is clear and a pale straw yellow color. Serum which appears cloudy is termed lipemic and denotes excess lipid material in the plasma. This may be the result of a pathological condition, or may be a normal artifact if the animal was not fasted before blood collection. Hemolyzed plasma can also occur as an artifact resulting from improper blood collection or processing. Hemolysis will also be evident in patients with conditions which cause the erythrocyte membrane to become unusually fragile. Yellowish, or icteric plasma is frequently seen in animals with liver disease or hemolytic anemia.

ERTHROCYTE SEDIMENTATION RATE (ESR)

The rate at which erythrocytes fall in their own plasma will be altered in certain disease states. Frequently, these alterations are the result of changes in the chemical structure of the erythrocyte membrane which then alter the physiology of the membrane. These changes usually cause the red blood cells to aggregate more readily.

The ESR is determined using a Wintrobe tube, filled as if for a macrohematocrit test. The tube is then set in a rack that holds the tube perpendicular to the table (Fig. 3-5). The rack is placed in an undisturbed location at controlled room temperature. After 60 minutes (20 minutes for equine), the level of the top of the column is read, utilizing the left hand scale on the tube. This measures the number of millimeters of fall for the specific time frame used.

The ESR will be affected by vibrations on the table surface and by variations in temperature in the lab. It will also be influenced by the total number of red cells in the sample. For this reason, it is necessary to correct the ESR value by subtracting the observed ESR from the expected ESR in a normal animal with the same PCV. Table 3-1 gives a chart of expected ESR values for various species and packed cell volumes. For example, a canine patient

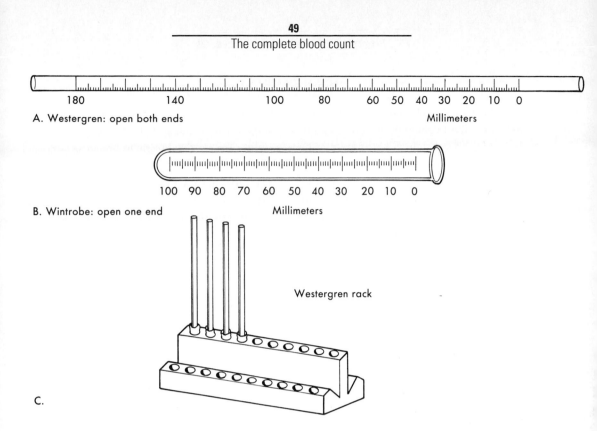

Fig. 3-5. Wintrobe and Westergen tubes for Erythrocyte Sedimentation Rate Measurement. (Powers, LW: *Diagnostic Hematology*, St. Louis, 1989, Mosby.)

with a PCV of 45% is expected to have an ESR of 5 mm. If the ESR is tested and found to be 12 mm, the corrected ESR for that patient would be recorded as +7 mm. Negative corrected ESR values may also occur, especially in animals with macrocytic erythrocytes.

TABLE 3-1
Erythrocyte sedimentation rate anticipated values

PVC%	Canine/feline (at 1 hour)	Equine (at 20 min)
10	79	86
15	64	80
20	49	70
25	36	60
30	26	47
35	16	28
40	10	11
45	5	2
50	0	0

HEMOGLOBIN

The earliest methodologies for hemoglobin measurement utilized a color standard sheet which was used to compare the color of a blood sample with a standard color, and this was correlated with a certain concentration of hemoglobin. These procedures can be performed either directly or indirectly. Direct matching involves placing a drop of whole blood on a piece of filter paper, allowing the drop to dry, and comparing the color with the standard. The indirect method requires that the red blood cells be lysed and then allowed to react in vitro with hydrochloric acid. This reaction forms the colored compound acid hematin, which can then be compared with color standards. Both of these methods are highly subjective, with a large probability of operator error.

Most procedures used for hemoglobin determination today use the cyanmethemoglobin methodology. The reagent used, Drabkin's solution, contains an agent to lyse the red blood cells (such as saponin) and an agent to oxidize the free hemoglobin and then convert it to cyanmethemoglobin (such as potassium ferricyanide).

To perform the procedure manually, a standard curve is prepared by diluting a commercially prepared solution of cyanmethemoglobin. This material is analyzed on the spectrophotometer and the percent of light absorbance or transmission is then plotted against the concentration of hemoglobin in each of the dilutions. Hemoglobin shows maximum absorbance at 540 nm.

A variety of automated and semiautomated instruments exist that are dedicated for hemoglobin measurement. One such instrument is the hemoglobinometer (Fig. 3-6). This is a portable, economical self-contained device that utilizes a small glass slide to hold a whole blood sample. The red blood cells in the sample are lysed with a wooden stick that contains hemolytic agents. The slide is then placed in the instrument and the operator matches the color of the light shown through the slide with a standard. This procedure can measure only the amount of oxyhemoglobin in the sample and has the potential for error in the subjective matching of the color. More recently, instruments such as the hemocue have been developed which eliminate the need for operator matching of color and read out the concentration of hemoglobin directly. These instruments are simple to use but require strict adherence to proper procedure to avoid operator error.

ERYTHROCYTE INDICES

The erythrocyte indices include the mean corpuscular volume (MCV), mean corpuscular hemoglobin (MCH) and mean corpuscular hemoglobin concentration (MCHC). These are calculated as part of the complete blood count. They can provide an objective and quantitative measure of the size of the red blood cells and their content of hemoglobin. The indices are especially useful in the classification of anemia. The accuracy of the calculations is dependent upon the individual accuracies of the total red cell count, the PCV, and the hemoglobin concentration.

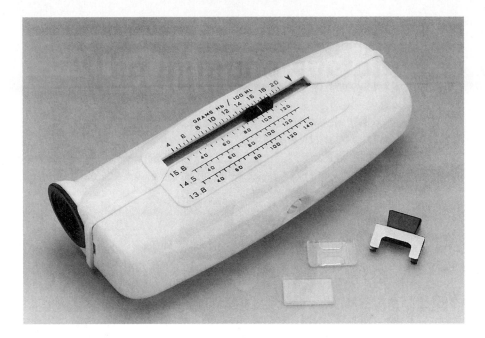

Fig. 3-6. The Hemoglobinometer is a dedicated instrument for hemoglobin measurement. (Photo courtesy of Leica Inc., 111 Deer Lake Rd., Deerfield, IL.)

Mean corpuscular volume refers to the average actual size of the red blood cells in circulation and is measured in femtoliters. MCV is calculated by multiplying the PCV value by 10 and dividing by the red blood cell count.

Mean corpuscular hemoglobin is a measure of the average weight of hemoglobin found in the circulating red blood cells and is measured in picograms. It is calculated by multiplying the hemoglobin concentration by 10 and then dividing by the total red blood cell count.

Mean corpuscular hemoglobin concentration is the ratio of the weight of hemoglobin per cell to the volume in which it is contained. MCHC is calculated by mutiplying the hemoglobin concentration by 100 and dividing by the PCV value. This result is expressed as a percent.

The MCHC utilizes only the PCV and Hb measurements. Both of these tests are associated with a greater degree of precision than the RBC count. Therefore, of the three indices, MCHC is the most accurate.

Values for erythrocyte indices should always be compared with morphology of the cells on the blood smear. For example, if microcytic cells are present on the smear, the MCV should be low.

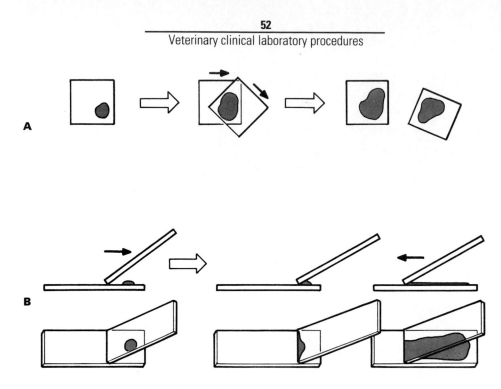

Fig. 3-7. Two commonly used methods of blood film preparation. **A**, Coverslip technique; **B**, wedge smear. (From Powers LW: *Diagnostic Hematology*, St. Louis, 1989, Mosby.)

THE DIFFERENTIAL BLOOD FILM

Examination of a prepared blood film can provide valuable information for the clinician. Such examination should include estimation of platelet numbers and evaluation of cellular morphology, as well as relative numbers of cell types.

Blood films can be prepared in several ways. The most commonly used methods are the coverslip preparation and the wedge smear (Fig. 3-7). Smears should always be made as soon as possible following blood collection, preferably within 15 minutes. Ideally, the drop of blood from the tip of the needle which has not been in contact with any anticoagulant should be used to make the smear. Always use new slides or coverslips and hold the slide by the edges only. This will avoid contamination of the slide with oils from the skin, which results in poor quality smears. The slide or coverslip should be dipped in alcohol and wiped dry before use.

A coverslip preparation is made by placing a small drop of blood on the center of one coverslip. A second coverslip is then placed diagonally on top of the first. The blood will spread through capillary action. The two coverslips are then gently pulled or slid apart using steady lateral motion just before the spread of blood is complete. The smears must be air dried by waving in the air and stained within one hour.

Wedge smears are prepared by placing a small drop of blood near one end of a clean glass slide. The edge of a second slide is used to spread the drop into an even film. Special "spreader" slides available for this purpose contain notched corners, or a regular glass slide can be used. The spreader slide is held at an angle of about 30° and brought into contact with the drop. Blood spreads along the edge of the slide by capillary action. The spreader slide is then pushed forward with a steady, firm, and even motion and a thin film of blood is formed. The slide must be immediately air dried and stained within one hour. The quality of this type of smear is dependent on the size of the drop, the angle of the spreader slide, and the downward pressure applied while spreading the film.

STAINING THE SMEAR

A number of commercial stains, referred to as Romanovsky stains, are available. Most are based on the Wright-Giemsa technique. This technique utilizes methylene blue dissolved in alcohol and eosin. The methylene blue is at an alkaline pH and has an affinity for the acidic components of the cell (nuclei). Eosin is at an acidic pH and stains the basic elements of the cell (hemoglobin and eosinophilic granules).

Some components of the cell can be stained only when the cell is in the living state. Since routine Wright's stain techniques fix the cell, vital dyes must be used. New methylene blue or brilliant cresyl blue stain the organelles and residual RNA found in the cytoplasm of living reticulocytes and Heinz bodies in erythrocytes.

Performing the differential

A good quality wedge smear will have a thick area near one end of the slide, which gradually tapers to a monolayer area and a feathered edge. In the monolayer area, the cells are evenly distributed, do not overlap, and show minimal distortion. The cells in the feathered edge area are usually greatly distorted and erratically distributed.

Place the smear on the microscope stage and examine under the scanning lens. Note the overall quality of the smear and the overall distribution of cells. Blood parasites and clumps of platelets may sometimes be concentrated in the feathered edge area of the smear, and these should be noted. With the low-power lens in place, locate the area just adjacent to the feathered edge where the monolayer begins. The count should proceed in an orderly fashion from this area inward toward the thick area of the smear. A variety of patterns for counting are acceptable, but the most commonly used method is shown in Fig. 3-8. With the oil immersion lens in place, count and classify at least one hundred leukocytes. A thorough evaluation of morphology and an estimation of platelet numbers must also be recorded.

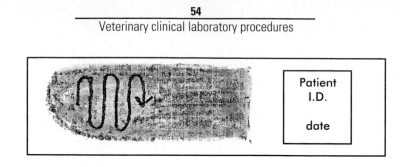

Fig. 3-8. Commonly used pattern for examination of differential blood film.

ERYTHROCYTE MORPHOLOGY

Of the cellular elements of blood, the erythrocyte (red blood cell) shows perhaps the greatest variation among mammalian species. It is vital that the technician be familiar with these normal variations in order for true abnormalities to be identified correctly. The proper identification of normal and abnormal red cell morphology is an important diagnostic tool that can provide the practitioner with invaluable information. Accurate morphologic evaluation can be made with the peripheral blood smear if the film is well-prepared and the examiner has had a reasonable amount of experience.

Red cell morphology can be defined as the appearance of the erythrocyte on a Wright's stained smear. The procedure for assessing morphology includes examining the smear under an oil immersion lens. This examination must be done in an area of the blood smear where the cells are randomly and evenly distributed and do not overlap.

ERYTHROCYTE ABNORMALITIES

Alteration in erythrocyte morphology occurs under numerous conditions. These variations generally fall into five categories: (1) variation in shape, (2) variation in color, (3) variation in size, (4) appearance of erythrocyte inclusions, and (5) variation in cell behavior.

Morphologic variations in size

Variation in erythrocyte diameter is found among normal individuals within a species and is termed *anisocytosis* (Table 3-2). It is often seen in young normal animals of most species and is marked in the normal bovine and rat of any age. These cells may be larger than normal (macrocytes), smaller than normal (microcytes), or a mixture of larger, smaller, and normal cells. Anisocytosis is a common finding in most anemias. The degree of anisocytosis increases with the severity of the anemia. Macrocytes usually represent newly released cells from the bone marrow or may be the result of a maturation defect, as in vitamin B_{12} deficiency. Microcytes are often the result of iron deficiency or malabsorption.

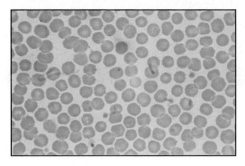

Normal feline erythrocytes

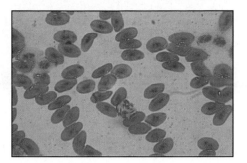

Normal avian blood cells

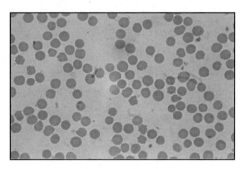

Anisocytosis in bovine blood

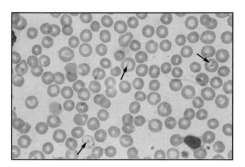

Target cells

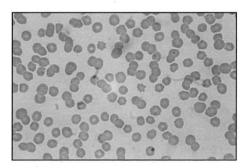

Mild rouleaux in equine blood

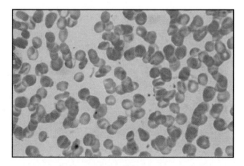

Autoagglutination in canine blood

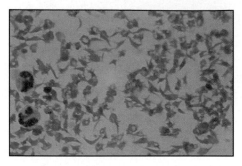

Sickled erythrocytes in deer blood

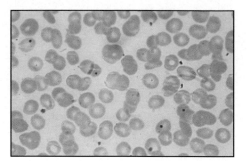

Howell-Jolly bodies

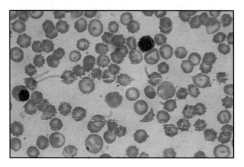

Immature erythrocytes—a nucleated erythrocyte and a rubricyte

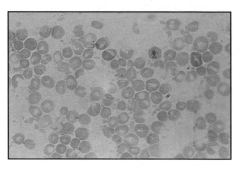

Reticulocytes

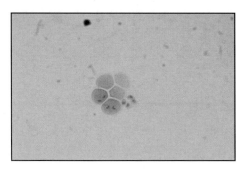

Babesia bovis

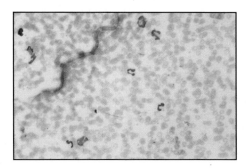

Microfilaria of *Dirofilaria immitis*

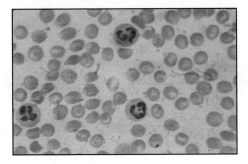

Normal neutrophils

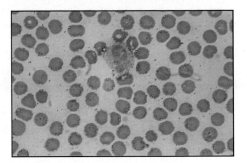

Neutrophil with toxic granulation

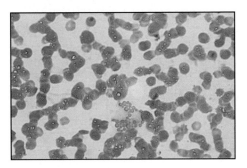

Equine eosinophil

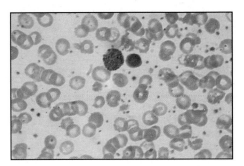

Basophil and small lymphocyte

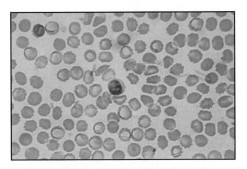

Canine lymphocyte

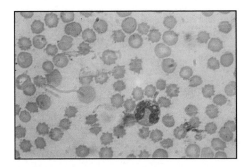

Canine monocyte

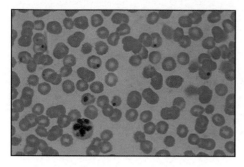

Hypersegmented neutrophil and distemper inclusion bodies

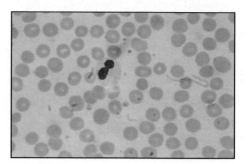

Pelger-Huet anomaly

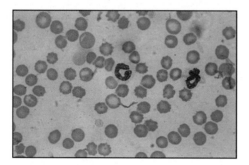

Neutrophilic band cells

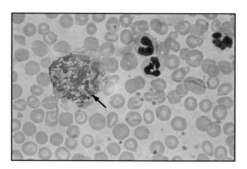

Smudge cell

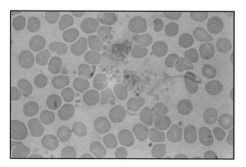

Clump of platelets

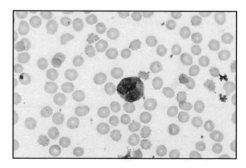

Kurloff body in leukocyte of a guinea pig

Morphologic variations in color

Erythrocytes which appear paler than normal on a routine Wright's stained blood smear are termed *hypochromic*. This condition is the manifestation of a reduced complement of hemoglobin within the cell. Hypochromasia is associated with iron deficiency anemia and lead poisoning and is often accompanied by microcytosis.

Cells which appear hypochromic may also result from a technical error during blood smear preparation. Excess pressure while making the smear may result in cells with "punched out" centers. These cells must be distinguished from anulocytes, which may also have this appearance. Unlike these punched out cells, true hypochromic cells have a gradual tapering of chromic material from the cell periphery to the paler region in the center.

Cells which appear darker than normal, or *hyperchromic*, give the appearance of being oversaturated with hemoglobin. Since the red blood cell has a fixed maximum hemoglobin-carrying capacity, such oversaturation cannot occur. These cells are usually microcytes or spherocytes.

Morphologic variations in shape

Poikilocytes are cells with abnormal shape and demonstrate species variation in that the origin of the alteration is often dependent on the species being examined. This cell type is abundant in most anemias.

Leptocytes are defined as cells with an increase in surface area relative to volume. They are best seen in thicker areas of the blood smear and are commonly of two types. *Target cells* are leptocytes with a central area of pigment surrounded by a clear zone and a dense ring of peripheral cytoplasm. A few may be seen in the normal blood smear and may also be associated with canine regenerative anemias, severe chronic organ disease, or inherited disorders. Target cells can also be produced as an artifact when the blood smear is

TABLE 3-2

Erythrocyte size

Species	Average diameter (μ)
Bovine	3.6 - 9.6
Ovine	3.5 - 6.0
Caprine	3.2 - 4.2
Porcine	4.0 - 8.0
Equine	5.6 - 8.0
Canine	6.7 - 7.3
Feline	5.4 - 6.3

dried too slowly or with the use of hypertonic fluids, such as salt-based anticoagulant. Leptocytes may also be in the form of *folded cells*, with a darkly stained "bar" of hemoglobin in the center as a result of the transverse fold. These are associated with bone marrow depression anemia, chronic infection, and splenic disease.

Spherocytes are cells with a decrease in surface area relative to cell volume and usually appear as hyperchromic microcytes. This condition is associated with hemolytic anemias and splenic disease.

Erythrocytes which are elliptical in shape are termed *ovalocytes* and are associated with macrocytic anemias. This abnormality can also be created as an artifact with the application of excessive pressure while preparing the blood smear. Ovalocytes are the predominant cell type found in the llama and other members of the camel family and do not indicate pathology in these species. They may also be found in the normal goat and sheep.

Acanthocytes have sharp, spine-like points that are irregularly spaced around the cell. These are often confused with crenated cells, which have rounded, evenly spaced projections. Crenation is usually an artifact resulting from dehydration of the cell due to slow drying of the blood smear and/or holding the blood at too high a temperature before making the smear. Acanthocytes are the result of damage to the erythrocyte membrane as would occur in uremia and liver disease.

Anulocytes appear bowl shaped as a result of a primary membrane defect which does not allow the flexibility necessary for the cell to return to its normal shape after passing through a capillary. The presence of this cell on a blood smear can also be an artifact resulting from the use of dirty slides. Anulocytes are seen in all animals with acute disease and in chronic disease of the canine.

Irregularly shaped fragments of erythrocytes, or *schistocytes*, are commonly seen in small numbers on most normal blood smears. In increased numbers, their presence would suggest hemolytic or immune-mediated anemia. In members of the deer family, the majority of the red blood cells may appear as schistocytes but are actually intact, sickled cells. Exposure to the environment causes this sickling phenomenon and is not necessarily indicative of pathology.

An erythrocyte with a linear rather than central area of pallor is termed a *stomatocyte* and is associated with inherited hemolytic anemia in the Alaskan Malamute breed of dog. This cell has a shortened life span and a regenerative response is usually evident in the patient.

Any erythrocyte abnormality should be correlated with other findings. For example, low MCH should be present when hypochromic cells are seen. Poor technique can often cause changes in erythrocytes that can mimic abnormal cells. These cells will frequently be present in only a small portion of the smear. True abnormalities will generally affect the majority of the cells on the smear. Any reported abnormality should be rated as to the percentage of cells involved. One commonly used system rates abnormalities on a scale from slight to +4, depending on the relative percentage of cells involved.

Variations in cell behavior

Rouleaux formation is characterized by cells that stick together in rows or chains. This may be produced as an artifact when blood is held too long before the smear is prepared. In a properly handled sample, the presence of rouleaux on the blood smear may suggest nutritional deficiency or multiple myeloma. In the equine, this condition often predominates and does not denote pathology.

Autoagglutination differs from rouleaux in that the cells are in three-dimensional clumps rather than rows. It can be distinguished from rouleaux by mixing the blood with saline. True autoagglutination will not disperse in saline and would usually indicate autoimmune hemolytic anemia.

OTHER ERYTHROCYTE ABNORMALITIES

Inclusion bodies

Poor technique, fixation artifacts, and precipitated stain can all be confused with inclusion bodies. An inclusion that appears refractile on a routinely stained blood film is most likely an artifact.

Reticulocytes are young anuclear cells which have retained some ribosomes, mitochondria, and/or endoplasmic reticulum. These cells usually appear polychromatophilic with Wright's stain and are often macrocytic. The use of a supravital stain (e.g., new methylene blue) is required for demonstration of blue granules or a network of blue filaments. The presence of reticulocytes in a blood smear from a normal individual is related to the characteristic erythrocyte life span of that species (Table 3-3). In species whose red blood cells have long life spans, there are few, if any, of these cells found in the normal patient. An increase in the relative percentage of reticulocytes in any species is an index of the regenerative activity of the blood and competency of the bone marrow.

TABLE 3-3

Erythrocyte life span

Species	Life span (days)
Bovine (adult)	160
(3 mos)	55
Equine	140-150
Porcine	62
Canine	107-115
Feline	68
Ovine	70-153
Caprine	125

Howell-Jolly bodies are remnants of nuclear material and appear as purple-blue inclusions, either singly or in pairs, which vary in size and location in the erythrocyte. This type of inclusion is often present in the normal canine, feline, and young porcine. They are also considered normal in the equine and appear as black bodies located eccentrically. In other species, Howell-Jolly bodies may accompany crisis stage anemia.

Other types of inclusion bodies found in erythrocytes require special handling to properly identify. *Heinz bodies* are inclusions that may affect up to 10% of the red blood cells of the normal feline. They may also be present in animals with certain hemolytic anemias. These bodies appear as pale areas within the cell on Wright's stained smears. They are composed of denatured hemoglobin and are best demonstrated with a vital stain (e.g., new methylene blue). With vital stains, they appear slightly refractile and are irregular in size and shape.

Generalized basophilia of the red blood cell may be due to inclusions that can be destroyed with the use of anticoagulants or fixation of the blood smear with methyl alcohol. If properly handled, *punctate basophilia* will appear as deep blue, coarse cytoplasmic granules that represent aggregations of iron-laden mitochondria and ribosomes. These cells are often hypochromic with routine staining procedures and indicate lead poisoning and other conditions that result in abnormal hemoglobin synthesis.

Nucleated erythrocytes can also occur in the normal patient, especially the young canine and porcine. In the adult animal, these cells denote an excessive demand for erythrocytes as would be found with leukemia and severe anemias. Since these are immature cells that have been released early, their presence gives an indication of the extent of bone marrow reaction.

Granules which appear as irregularly contoured, bluish-black inclusions in Wright's stained preparations are *siderotic granules* and consist of small particles of nonhemoglobin iron and iron-laden mitochondria. These are often confused with punctate basophilia and may be differentiated with special staining compounds such as, Prussian blue. Siderotic granules are associated with defects in hemoglobin synthesis, iron toxicity, and hypochromic anemias.

LEUKOCYTE MORPHOLOGY

A properly performed differential blood cell count contains information that not only enumerates the various cell types but describes them in morphologic terms. The identification of both normal and abnormal leukocytes can be complicated unless the technician is familiar with the distinct morphologic variations of the leukocytes of a given species.

Morphologic variation in leukocytes

Morphologic variation in leukocytes can be due to a number of conditions, which may be pathologic, nonpathologic, or reactive. Pathologic cells show abnormalities in appearance and/or function and indicate an abnormal response to a stimulus or defect. These always result in physiologic impairment in the animal. Reactive leukocytes will show marked alteration in appearance but are functioning normally as a response to a disease process.

Nonpathologic leukocytes may also be found. Although these cell show alteration in appearance, their function is unaffected.

The more common morphologic variations of leukocytes can be divided into several categories on the basis of the nature of the alteration: (1) nuclear variation, (2) cytoplasmic inclusions, (3) parasites, (4) juvenile forms, and (5) miscellaneous forms.

NUCLEAR VARIATION

A nucleus which contains six or more lobes is said to be hypersegmented. This occurs most frequently in the neutrophil but can be seen in any granulocyte. The cytoplasm is normal in appearance and function. This condition is thought to be a result of aging processes, which normally occur in tissue spaces rather than in peripheral circulation, and is considered pathologic. In domestic animals, hypersegmented cells are a common finding in chronic infection, folic acid deficiency, pernicious anemia, and in animals taking steroids. Hyper-segmentation may also be produced as an artifact when the blood sample is allowed to sit for several hours before the smear is prepared.

The giant neutrophil is a hypersegmented cell that has an average diameter greater than 16 μm. This denotes defective maturation and is associated with the recovery phase of feline panleukopenia.

Hyposegmentation involves a nucleus which contains less than three lobes and may be round, peanut-shaped, band, or bilobed. The condition, termed Pelger-Huet anomaly, is known to occur in dogs and rabbits. The chromatin material often appears pyknotic. This abnormality occurs with severe infection and burns and is often found in animals taking sulfa drugs.

Barr bodies are drumstick-like projections that are attached to the lobe of the neu-trophil nucleus by a single narrow stalk. These represent the inactivated X chromosome in the female and are not significant unless there is more than one per cell or the patient is a male.

Karyorrhexis and karyolysis describe a leukocyte nucleus which appears condensed, fragmented, or lysed. This condition is an artifact created with the use of oxalate anticoagu-lants. Oxalates result in immediate and marked deterioration of white blood cells and make it impossible to accurately describe cell morphology.

CYTOPLASMIC VARIATION

Döhle bodies are small, gray-blue, irregular patches of cytoplasm usually found near the cell periphery. Although seen primarily in neutrophils, they can be in any of the granulo-cytes. These patches are composed of ribosomes and denote immature cytoplasm. Döhle bodies occur most commonly in the cat and may be seen in animals with severe bacterial infection and some severe viral diseases.

Vacuolization of lymphocytes and/or neutrophils is associated with septicemia, but can also be produced as an artifact if the blood is held too long in anticoagulant (especially EDTA) before the smear is made.

Chediak-Higashi anomaly is characterized by large, coarse, eosinophilic, irregular granules in the cytoplasm of granulocytes and monocytes. In the lymphocyte, the granules are often large and azurophilic. These granules represent abnormal lysosomes and are associated with lymphadenopathy and recurrent infection. In contrast, a fine, eosinophilic granulation of the neutrophil is an inherited anomaly in some domestic felines and is not associated with pathology. This anomaly is also found in the rabbit and guinea pig. Kurloff bodies are also found in the guinea pig and appear as eosinophilic inclusions in neutrophils. These are most numerous in the female guinea pig and are markedly increased during pregnancy.

Distemper inclusion bodies are a rare finding on the blood smear but may be seen in any of the leukocytes or erythrocytes. These are composed of viral nucleocapsids and stain pale blue or red. Due to the small numbers of inclusions normally found, it is easiest to demonstrate these with a buffy coat smear.

Toxic granulation is characterized by the presence of numerous large granules in the cytoplasm of both segmented and band neutrophils. The granules range in color from purplish-blue to red and indicate severe infection. This condition occurs most frequently in the equine but is seen in all species in severe infections and other toxic states.

Blood parasites

A number of parasites can be found both intracellularly and free of cells on the peripheral blood smear. Many of these are parasites of the cells in which they occur, while others are being transported to other parts of the body via the circulatory system, or are present in the bloodstream as part of their life cycle but cause no pathology there.

Anaplasma species is a Rickettsial parasite of the bovine. It usually appears as a small round structure near the cell periphery and may be in pairs. If supravital stains are used, the tails and loop-like appendages of the parasite may be seen. Anaplasma organisms often have a halo and are usually uniform in size.

A number of *Babesia* species are parasites of mammals, primarily the bovine, equine, and canine. These parasites appear as round, oval, or tear-shaped bodies which can occur singly, in pairs, or in multiples of two. If in pairs, the two are connected by an eosinophilic strand. The size of the organisms varies depending on the species and, in the equine, they often form tetrads. Infected cells are often macrocytic and are best seen in the feathered edge area of the smear.

Bovine, ovine, porcine, and some laboratory animals can be infected with the *Eperythrozoon* species parasite. These parasites form ring-like structures and can occur as cocci, rods, and budding forms. They may also be seen free of cells.

One of the most commonly observed parasites of canine and feline species is *Haemobartonella*, which is difficult to find on a peripheral blood smear. When present, it appears in many forms on the erythrocyte, including cocci, rods, and bows, and may occur singly or in pairs. The affected cells are usually macrocytic.

Plasmodium species attacks the red blood cells of a number of mammalian species, such as rodents, ruminants, and primates, including man. Many stages of the parasite can occur in the cell. Earlier stages often appear as signet rings, while mature forms are usually individual bodies which completely fill the enlarged cell.

Another parasite which is rarely found on the blood smear is the *Theileria* species. This organism attacks the red blood cells of bovine, ovine, caprine, and deer families and appears as small bodies with deeply stained nuclei and basophilic cytoplasm. It may also be seen in lymphocytes.

Feline erythrocytes may be infected with the *Cytauxzoon* organism. These parasites appear as single, round to slightly oval bodies with a small, peripheral dark purple nucleus. Often, less than 5% of the red blood cells will be involved.

Trypanosoma species, while not specifically a "blood" parasite, can sometimes be found on the blood smear. These are large, broad parasites with flagella usually visible and a large kinetoplast.

Microfilaria of *Dirofilaria* species, the causative agent of canine heartworm disease, can often be found on the blood smear and are easiest to see in the feathered edge area of the blood smear.

Histoplasma species are sometimes found in the canine leukocyte and may be in the nucleus, cytoplasm, or both. Their staining characteristics are unpredictable, but are usually seen as a dark nucleus with a thin, clear capsule.

Ehrlichia parasites are primarily found in lymphocytes but may be seen in the neutrophil or monocyte. These are often seen in conjunction with *Brucella canis* and are best demonstrated with a buffy coat smear due to the generally low parasite numbers.

Although primarily in muscle, the gametocyte stage of *Hepatozoon* species may appear faintly stained in the neutrophil and monocyte.

Toxoplasma parasites are of concern in both small and food animal practice. The organism is elongated, rounded at one end, and tapering slightly at the other. These are often crescentic but may vary to extreme ovoid forms. A well-defined nucleus and small red staining paranuclear body may be seen. The parasite is found in all tissue spaces and less often in peripheral circulation.

JUVENILE AND MISCELLANEOUS FORMS

Band cells are commonly seen in small numbers in most species except the bovine. The nucleus appears as a curved band with parallel sides. Large numbers of this cell type, when accompanied by an increased total white blood cell count, indicate a regenerative shift. Regenerative shifts often indicate that an animal is responding appropriately to a disease condition. Bone marrow activity increases and immature cells are released from the bone marrow in an attempt to combat the disease. Large numbers of band cells found in conjunction with a normal or decreased total leukocyte count indicate a degenerative shift. Metamyelocytes are immature forms of leukocyte that are not normally seen in the peripheral blood of any species. The cytoplasm may contain neutrophilic, eosinophilic, or basophilic granules. The presence of this cell type denotes a severe disease process.

Plasma cells are derived from the B-Lymphocyte and are the major cellular source of immunoglobulins. Although the cell itself is not abnormal, its presence in the peripheral circulation is uncommon and is associated with viral infection and hypersensitivity reactions. An eccentric nucleus with chromatin material arranged like the spokes of a wheel, abundant dark blue cytoplasm and cytoplasmic vacuoles are characteristic.

Smudge cells (also called basket cells) are degenerative cells that have ruptured. The nucleus appears as a pale staining smear lacking shape or form. These are usually an artifact produced with excessive pressure when making the smear and in small numbers are not considered significant. The number of basket cells per one hundred white blood cells should be reported along with the differential count. Basket cells are commonly seen when old blood samples are used for analysis.

Mast cells are connective tissue cells with granules that stain metachromatically. The granules tend to vary in size but are usually uniform within a given cell. Low numbers of this cell type may be seen with many different inflammatory diseases, such as parvovirus infection. Increased numbers of mast cells in circulation may indicate mast cell leukemia. In the rabbit, trauma at the venipuncture site may also result in increased mast cells.

Other types of atypical cells are seen in many types of leukemia. These cells are primarily blast cells and often appear very similar morphologically. Special staining techniques and/or referral to a specialist may be needed to positively identify the cell line involved.

Absolute values

The differential blood film provides a relative measure of the different types of leukocytes present in the blood. If the percentage of one cell type is increased, this can be due either to a real increase or a decrease in another cell type. Absolute values for leukocytes can be used to distinguish between these two cases. The absolute value is calculated by multiplying the percentage of each cell type by the total leukocyte count. For example, if 50% neutrophils are present in a sample with a white blood cell count of 48,000, then the absolute neutrophil value is 24,000. A relative neutrophil count of 50% represents a decrease. However, the absolute value in this case is actually quite high.

THROMBOCYTES

The evaluation of thrombocytes, or platelets, is a part of all routine differential white blood cell counts.

APPEARANCE

Platelets vary in size from 1 to 4 μm and may have multiple pointed projections. They are generally round, oval, or spindle-shaped and stain pale blue with purplish granules. They tend to stick together, and any blood smear must be examined for the presence of large clumps of platelets, often found in the feathered edge area of the smear.

MORPHOLOGIC VARIATION

Giant platelets, can occur in any species but are most commonly seen in the feline and bovine. There is little or no variation in the morphology of mammalian thrombocytes.

THROMBOCYTE COUNT

An indirect measure of the number of thrombocytes can be made by examining the peripheral blood film. The number of platelets in ten oil immersion fields is counted and averaged. In a normal patient, the number of thrombocytes averaged over ten oil immersion fields should be between 7 and 21. A value in this range can be recorded as a platelet estimate of 'normal.'

A second indirect measure is to count the number of thrombocytes on the blood film for each 100 leukocytes. The thrombocyte count can be estimated with the following calculation:

$$\frac{\text{No. of thrombocytes}}{100 \text{ leukocytes}} \times \frac{\text{Total WBC count}}{\text{mm}^3} = \text{Total thrombocytes/mm}^3$$

Direct platelet measurements are performed in a manner similar to that for red and white blood cells counts. Thrombocyte counts are generally more difficult as a result of their small size and their ready agglutination. They also tend to disintegrate rapidly and will easily adhere to surfaces. Blood for thrombocyte counts should be drawn in a plastic syringe and treated with EDTA. An appropriate diluent which can prevent aggregation of the platelets, preserve their integrity, and lyse the red blood cells should be chosen. One common commercially available diluent is the Rees-Ecker, which also stains the platelets. The Unopette system also has a reservoir available which is designed specifically for thrombocyte counts. In general, ten squares in the super square of the hemocytometer should be counted on each side. Platelets usually appear light blue, may be vibrating, and are round and refractile. The same calculation used for erythrocyte and leukocyte counts is utilized for direct thrombocyte counts.

RETICULOCYTE COUNTS

Enumeration of the reticulocytes on a differential blood film can provide valuable information to the clinician regarding the type of any anemia present and whether the bone marrow is properly responding to the condition. Vital stain (e.g., new methylene blue) is required and two methods exist, the slide method and the tube method.

The tube method requires three drops of vital stain that is mixed, filtered, and placed in a small test tube. Two drops of a well-mixed EDTA treated sample are added to the tube. The tube is gently mixed for three to five minutes. Three thin smears are prepared from this mixture. The smear is examined and the monolayer located. Using the oil immersion lens, the number of reticulocytes and total erythrocytes is counted. After one thousand erythrocytes have been counted, the percent of reticulocytes is calculated as follows:

$$\frac{\text{\# of reticulocytes}}{1000 \text{ RBCs}} \times 100 = \% \text{ reticulocytes}$$

The reticulocyte count can also be performed with the slide method. One drop of vital stain is placed at the end of a slide and allowed to dry. A drop of blood is then added to the stain and mixed. The slide is left undisturbed for one minute and then the mixture is smeared across the slide. The count and calculation is completed as for the tube method.

ERYTHROCYTE FRAGILITY

In certain disease conditions, the erythrocyte may demonstrate alteration in its resistance to hemolysis. Reticulocytes are more resistant to lysis than mature red blood cells. Certain immune-mediated hemolytic diseases may increase the fragility of the erythrocyte (i.e., the cell lyses more readily).

Erythrocyte fragility is easily measured with the Unopette RBC osmotic fragility test kit. This kit contains ten reservoirs, each with a different concentration of buffered saline solution. The saline concentrations range from 0.85%, which is isotonic to erythrocytes, to 0.00%, which is hypotonic. In the hypotonic solutions, the erythrocytes will take up water and eventually lyse. Hemoglobin is released into the solution by the lysed cells, causing a color change in the solution. The absorbance (Abs) of each solution is measured in the spectrophotometer. The percent hemolysis in each solution is calculated as follows:

$$\% \text{ Hemolysis} = \frac{\text{Abs of solution} - \text{Abs of .85\% solution}}{\text{Abs of 0.00\% solution} - \text{Abs of .85\% solution}} \times 100$$

These percentages are then plotted on straight line graph paper against the concentration of saline in each solution. In normal animals, the graph should represent a sigmoid curve (Fig. 3-9).

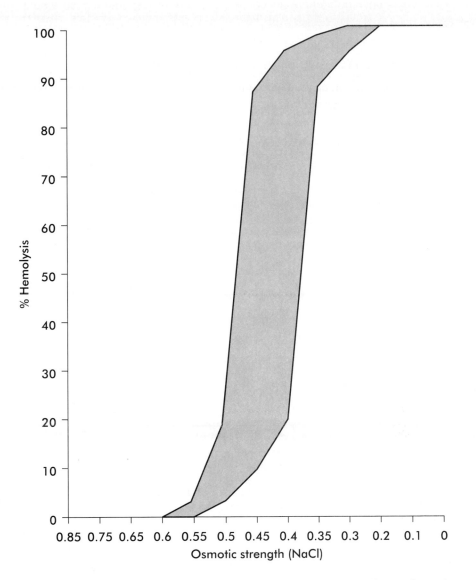

Fig. 3-9. Osmotic fragility curve—*shaded area* shows normal range for canine.

KEY POINTS

1. The minimum tests required for a complete blood count are erythrocyte and leukocyte counts, differential cell count, PCV, and hemoglobin measurement.

2. Erythrocyte and leukocyte counts are performed on a diluted blood sample with a hemocytometer.

3. Polycythemia is an increase in the number of circulating erythrocytes.

4. Splenic contraction in an animal that is stressed during blood collection will often result in transient polycythemia.

5. Anemia is a reduction in the oxygen-carrying capacity of blood due to a decrease in number of erythrocytes and/or hemoglobin concentration.

6. The packed cell volume is determined by centrifugation of an anticoagulated blood sample.

7. The macrohematocrit method is more accurate than the microhematocrit method for determination of packed cell volume.

8. The ESR represents the rate at which erythrocytes fall in their own plasma under controlled conditions.

9. The ESR will be influenced by the total red cell mass and must be corrected by subtracting the observed ESR from the ESR expected with the same PCV.

10. Both the direct matching and acid hematin methods for hemoglobin determination are subjective tests which require visual matching of color standards.

11. The cyanmethemoglobin procedure for hemoglobin determination measures all forms of hemoglobin in the blood sample.

12. Erythrocyte indices are calculated from the red cell count, PCV, and hemoglobin measurements.

13. Erythrocyte indices provide a measurement of the average volume and hemoglobin concentration of the erythrocytes and are used in the classification of anemias.

14. The differential blood smear is used to estimate the relative percentages of each type of blood leukocyte, to estimate platelet numbers, and to evaluate cell morphology.

15. Differentials are performed only in the monolayer area where cells are evenly and randomly distributed and do not overlap.

16. Alterations in erythrocyte morphology include variations in color, shape, size, cell behavior, and appearance of inclusions.

17. Erythrocyte abnormalities should always be correlated with other findings.

18. Reticulocytes are anuclear, immature erythrocytes that appear macrocytic and polychromatophilic on Wright's stained smears.

19. Most erythrocyte inclusions represent remnants of organelles.

20. Morphologic variation in leukocytes may affect the cell nucleus, cytoplasm, or both.

21. Absolute leukocyte values provide a more reliable indicator of the actual numbers of each cell type than relative counts taken from the differential.

22. Platelet numbers can be estimated indirectly from the blood smear.

23. Reticulocyte counts are performed on a blood smear stained with a supravital stain.

24. Osmotic fragility is a measure of the susceptibility of the erythrocyte to lysis in solutions of varying osmotic concentration.

REVIEW QUESTIONS

1. True or False. The diluent used for erythrocyte counts must be hypotonic for erythrocytes.
2. Write the general equation for calculation of cell counts.
3. List three nonpathologic causes of real or apparent polycythemia.
4. Define anemia.
5. List the layers formed, in order, in the hematocrit tube following centrifugation for packed cell volume.
6. Of what does the buffy coat consist?
7. A red tinged buffy coat indicates the presence of _____.
8. Describe the principle behind the cyanmethemoglobin procedure for hemoglobin determination.
9. Blood parasites are sometimes found in the _____ area of the blood smear.
10. Variation in erythrocyte size is termed _____.
11. Erythrocytes with a larger than normal area of central pallor are referred to as _____.
12. List the types of poikilocytic cells that may be identified on the blood smear.
13. A large polychromatophilic erythrocyte on a Wright's stained smear is most likely a _____.
14. Large numbers of band cells accompanying an increase in total leukocyte numbers is referred to as a _____.
15. Enumeration of reticulocytes requires a blood smear stained with _____.
16. Describe the general procedure for erythrocyte fragility testing.

ANSWERS TO REVIEW QUESTIONS

1. False. The diluent used for erythrocyte counts must be isotonic. Hypotonic diluents will lyse erythrocytes.

2. Cell counts $= \dfrac{\text{Avg. no. of cells per hemocytometer grid}}{\text{dilution ratio} \times \text{vol. of one square} \times \text{no. of squares counted}}$

3. Real or apparent polycythemia may be caused by dehydration, splenic contraction, and high altitudes.

4. Anemia is a reduction in the oxygen-carrying capacity of the blood due to a decrease in number of red blood cells and/or hemoglobin concentration.

5. The layers formed, in order, in the hematocrit tube following centrifugation for packed cell volume are the packed red cells, the buffy coat, and the blood plasma.

6. The buffy coat consists of leukocytes, thrombocytes, and sometimes nucleated red blood cells.

7. A red tinged buffy coat indicates the presence of nucleated red blood cells.

8. A lysing agent is used to hemolyze the erythrocytes. The freed hemoglobin reacts with potassium ferricyanide to form the colored compound cyanmethemoglobin.

9. Blood parasites are sometimes found in the feathered edge area of the blood smear.

10. Variation in erythrocyte size is termed anisocytosis.

11. Erythrocytes with a larger than normal area of central pallor are referred to as hypochromic.

12. The types of poikilocytic cells that may be identified on the blood smear include leptocytes, spherocytes, ovalocytes, acanthocytes, anulocytes, schistocytes, and stomatocytes.

13. A large polychromatophilic erythrocyte on a Wright's stained smear is most likely a reticulocyte.

14. Large numbers of band cells accompanying an increase in total leukocyte numbers is referred to as a regenerative shift.

15. Enumeration of reticulocytes requires a blood smear stained with a supravital stain, such as new methylene blue.

16. Erythrocyte fragility testing requires hypotonic solutions of varying osmotic concentration. Erythrocytes are introduced into the solutions that will be lysed. The absorbance of each solution is measured and the percent hemolysis in each solution is calculated. Percent hemolysis is plotted on straight line graph paper against concentration of each of the solutions.

SELECTED READING

Powers LW: *Diagnostic Hematology: clinical and technical principles.* St. Louis, 1989, CV Mosby Co.

Coles EH: *Veterinary Clinical Pathology*, ed 4. Philadelphia, 1986, WB Saunders.

Schalm OW, Jain NC, Carroll EJ: *Veterinary Hematology*, ed 3. Philadelphia, 1975, Lea & Febiger.

Benjamin M: *Outline of Veterinary Clinical Pathology*, ed 3. Ames, IA, 1978, Iowa State University Press.

Bauer JD: *Clinical Laboratory Methods*, ed 9. St. Louis, 1982, CV Mosby Co.

Dacie JV, Lewis SM: *Practical Hematology*, ed 6. New York, 1984, Churchill Livingstone.

Rich LJ: *The Morphology of Canine & Feline Blood Cells.* St. Louis, 1976, Ralston Purina Co.

Dein FJ: *Laboratory Manual of Avian Hematology.* East Northport, NY, 1984, Association of Avian Veterinarians.

Schalm OW: *Manual of Feline and Canine Hematology.* Santa Barbara, CA, 1980, Veterinary Practice Publishing Co.

Schalm OW: *Manual of Equine Hematology.* Santa Barbara, CA, 1984, Veterinary Practice Publishing Co.

Schalm OW: *Manual of Bovine Hematology.* Santa Barbara, CA, 1984, Veterinary Practice Publishing Co.

Blood coagulation

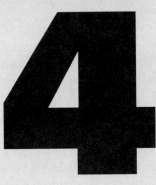

PERFORMANCE OBJECTIVES
After completion of this chapter, the student will:

Define hemostasis.

Describe the role of thrombocytes in the blood coagulation mechanism.

Identify the coagulation factors and describe the role of each.

Diagram the blood coagulation pathways.

List the factors which can contribute to hemostatic defects.

Describe the procedure for direct enumeration of thrombocytes.

List the coagulation tests and identify which
portion(s) of the coagulation pathway are evaluated with each.

Describe the procedure for performing the Activated Clotting Time test.

T he ability to maintain the integrity of blood vessels and fluid is termed hemostasis. An evaluation of hemostatic mechanisms should be included as part of most routine presurgical workups. An understanding of the mechanisms involved in hemostasis is crucial to the selection of appropriate test methodologies.

Blood coagulation proceeds through both a mechanical and a chemical phase. Mechanical hemostasis involves constriction of blood vessels and aggregation of platelets and is triggered by blood vessel injury. This injury results in the release of chemicals by the blood vessel endothelium which cause constriction of the vessel. If the surrounding tissue is also damaged, tissue cells will release similar chemicals to constrict the tissue. Platelets are attracted to the charged surface of the exposed basement membrane and begin to aggregate and adhere to the site of the injury. This aggregation results in the formation of a hemostatic plug over the damaged area. Platelet aggregation occurs very rapidly, usually within 30 seconds after injury. As platelets attach to the surface and to each other, they undergo a series of morphologic and biochemical changes. These changes serve to activate the platelets for their role in the chemical phase of hemostasis.

Chemical hemostasis is referred to as the coagulation cascade and involves numerous chemical constituents of the blood plasma as well as chemical agents released by platelets and damaged cells. The cascade reactions may be triggered through either an extrinsic or intrinsic pathway. Both pathways then culminate in a common pathway. A list of the coagulation factors involved may be found in Table 4-1.

The extrinsic pathway is activated quickly and may be completed in as little as 15 seconds. In the presence of tissue thromboplastin (factor III) which is released by damaged cells, factor VII is activated and this activates factor X. Calcium (factor IV) and specific phospholipids are also required for these reactions. Activated factor X is thus prepared for its role in the common pathway.

TABLE 4-1

Blood coagulation factors

Designation	Synonym
Factor I	Fibrinogen
Factor II	Prothrombin
Factor III	Tissue thromboplastin
Factor IV	Calcium
Factor V	Proaccelerin
Factor VII	Proconvertin
Factor VIII	Anithemophilic factor
Factor IX	Christmas factor, Plasma thromboplastin
Factor X	Stuart-Prower factor
Factor XI	Plasma thromboplastin antecedent
Factor XII	Hageman factor
Factor XIII	Fibrin-stabilizing factor

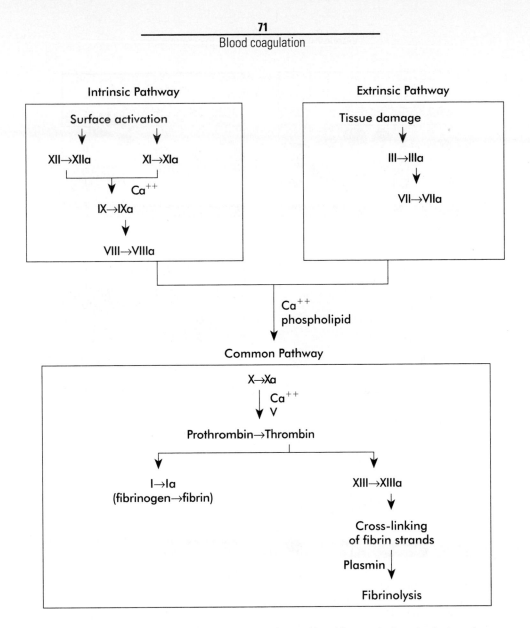

Fig. 4-1. The Blood Coagulation Cascade can be triggered by either extrinsic or intrinsic pathways.

The intrinsic pathway is triggered by the contact of factors XI and XII with the charged surface of the damaged blood vessel endothelium. Factors VIII and IX are then activated, again in the presence of calcium and phospholipid. With the presence of platelet factor 3, the activated factor VIII/IX complex serves to activate factor X for its role in the common pathway.

The reactions of the coagulation cascade are complex and a number of additional interactions and intermediate steps exist within the pathways. A complete discussion of these reactions is beyond the scope of this text. Fig. 4-1 summarizes the reactions of the various pathways.

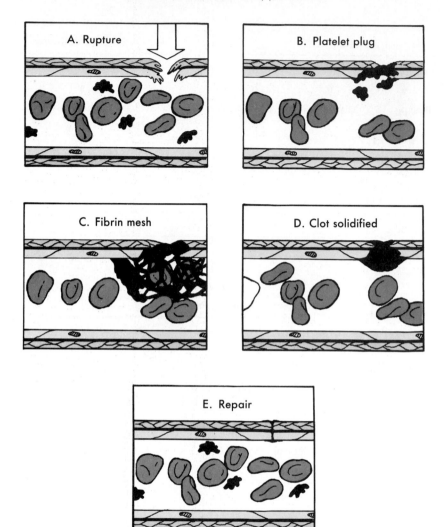

Fig. 4-2. Formation and retraction of a fibrin clot. (From Powers LW: *Diagnostic Hematology*, St. Louis, 1989, Mosby)

The activation of factor X through either pathway results in the generation of thrombin from its precursor, prothrombin. This occurs as a result of a series of reactions which also involve factor V, calcium, and platelet factor 3. Thrombin then serves as the activator for factor XIII and factor I (fibrinogen). Fibrinogen is converted to fibrin which then aggregates as numerous fibrin strands over the damaged area. Factor XIII serves to cross link and stabilize these strands.

TABLE 4-2

Congenital and hereditary coagulation defects

Disease	Inheritance pattern	Animals affected
Hemophilia A (factor VIII defect or deficiency)	Sex-linked Recessive	All
Hemophilia B (factor IX deficiency) (Christmas disease)	Sex-linked	Terriers Schnauzers Poodles
Factor VII deficiency	Autosomal incomplete dominance	Beagles
Factor X deficiency	Autosomal/recessive incomplete dominance	Cocker Spaniels
vonWillebrand's disease	Autosomal incomplete dominance	Canines—especially Dobermans, German Shepherds, Golden Retrievers
Factor XI deficiency	Autosomal recessive	Spaniels; cattle
Platelet abnormalities (defects in number or function)	Sex-linked or Autosomal	Hounds

The final stage in the hemostatic mechanism is the restoration of normal blood vessel integrity by the degradation of the fibrin clot. This involves the molecule plasmin which is activated by several factors and serves to constrict and fragment the fibrin clot (Fig. 4-2).

HEMOSTATIC DEFECTS

Pathologic changes in coagulation ability may be a primary disease condition or occur secondary to some other disease process. A complete physical examination and thorough patient history will assist the clinician in pinpointing the nature of the defect. Bleeding disorders in a young animal are most likely inherited defects (Table 4-2). If a bleeding disorder is detected for the first time in an adult animal, acquired defects are more likely.

Types of hemorrhage

Spontaneous hemorrhage into body cavities is seen in severe cases of coagulation defects. This type of large hemorrhage is common when a defect within the chemical phase of hemostasis is present. Disorders within the mechanical phase usually result in small bleeding episodes. Purpura, which represents small hemorrhage in skin and mucous membranes, is a common finding. Hemorrhage into the retina of the eye may be present. Blood in the urine (hematuria) or feces (melena) is occasionally seen.

Primary coagulation defects

Hereditary abnormalities which impair coagulation include a number of factor deficiencies. Such deficiencies may be either quantitative or functional. Frequently, a specific factor deficiency is associated with a specific animal or breed. Most of these diseases are quite rare. One notable exception is vonWillebrand's disease (vWD), the most common inherited bleeding disorder. This disease involves a functional deficiency of vonWillebrand's factor, a plasma protein which aids in the initial adherence of platelets to the blood vessel endothelium and helps initiate the intrinsic pathway. Animals with vWD are unable to synthesize an adequate amount of a physiologically active form of vonWillebrand's factor. Three different types of vWD have been described based on their different patterns of inheritance and resulting differences in the amount and type of abnormal vonWillebrand's factor produced. Most canine vWD is Type I which is inherited as an autosomal defect with incomplete dominance. This disorder is especially common in Doberman Pinschers and is usually lethal if homozygous. vWD has been described in 54 dog breeds and has also been reported in pigs. vonWillebrand's factor is associated with a component of factor VIII. Animals with vWD frequently have a corresponding reduction in factor VIII activity. Deficiencies of factor VIII cause the disease hemophilia A. The defect, inherited as an X-linked recessive disorder, is seen in most breeds of dogs and in cats.

Secondary coagulation defects

Acquired abnormalities are more common than hereditary coagulation defects and usually occur secondary to some other disease process. Since the liver is the primary site for synthesis of most coagulation factors, any disease which is characterized by impaired liver function can result in deficiencies of coagulation factors. Vitamin K is required for synthesis of factors II, VII, IX, and X. Inadequate consumption or malabsorption of vitamin K can therefore also cause bleeding disorders. The toxicity associated with ingestion of rodenticides (e.g., warfarin) is related to the inhibition of vitamin K function by these compounds and the resulting deficiency of coagulation factors. Ingestion of natural anticoagulants, such as those found in moldy sweet clover, also acts to inhibit vitamin K function. Ingestion of certain drugs can also have a negative effect on blood coagulation. Sulfa drugs and aspirin act to inhibit proper blood coagulation. Aspirin, in particular, should be avoided in patients prior to surgery. Aspirin acts to permanently inhibit platelet adherence, and its effects can be seen for 5 to 10 days after ingestion.

Abnormally low platelet count is termed thrombocytopenia. This condition may be caused by decreased production and associated with bone marrow abnormality or may be the result of hereditary or congenital defects. Administration of estradiol can result in bleeding defects due to bone marrow suppression. Certain viral and rickettsial agents may also result in thrombocytopenia. The range of normal thrombocyte values is quite large (150 to 400 $\times$ $10^3/\mu l$). However, the level within an individual animal is relatively constant. Counts less than $100 \times 10^3/\mu l$ signify thrombocytopenia. Counts less than $40 \times 10^3/\mu l$ usually indicate a significant disorder. Increased destruction or consumption of platlets can also be a cause of low platelet counts. Certain autoimmune diseases may involve the production of antibodies to platelets which result in increased destruction. Disseminated intravascular coagulation (DIC) often occurs secondarily to a number of disease conditions and is accompanied by a decrease in thrombocyte counts. DIC involves the formation of numerous clots throughout the body which deplete platelets, as well as coagulation factors. Thrombocytosis, or abnormally high platelet count, is rare but may be seen associated with regenerative anemias and in animals that have been splenectomized.

HEMOSTATIC EVALUATIONS

Hemostatic evaluations are necessary to detect the presence and cause of any pathologic changes in hemostatic ability. Laboratory tests can be chosen which evaluate specific portions of the coagulation cascade or the mechanical phase of hemostasis.

Sample collection and handling

Improper sample collection can invalidate laboratory results of coagulation testing. Platelets will aggregate on rough surfaces and this can result in initiation of the coagulation pathway in vitro. Platelets are less likely to aggregate on the smooth surfaces of plastic or siliconized glass tubes.

EDTA is suitable as an anticoagulant when thrombocyte counts are required, but it can inhibit platelet function. The preferred anticoagulants for most coagulation testing are citrates or oxalates. The plasma sample is obtained by centrifugation and tested immediately. If testing is to be delayed, the plasma should be frozen. Samples for platelet testing must be kept at room temperature and tested within 2 hours. Exposure to heat or cold will alter platelet shape and inhibit proper function. Platelet-poor plasma is obtained by centrifuging the sample at 1000 G for 15 minutes and is used for most coagulation testing. Platelet-rich plasma can be harvested following centrifugation at 1000 G for 5 to 10 minutes. Critical tests of platelet function will require platelet-rich plasma samples.

Thrombocyte count

Methods to estimate platelet numbers were described in Chapter 3. When coagulation disorders are suspected, a direct thrombocyte count should be performed.

Evaluation of platelet numbers may be accomplished by manual or automated methods. Manual counts are made using a hemocytometer and properly collected and diluted blood sample. Specific diluents for platelet counts are commercially available. A Unopette reservoir for platelet determinations is also available. The Unopette system diluent lyses the red blood cells, while leaving the thrombocytes and leukocytes intact. Once charged with the diluted blood sample, the hemocytometer must be placed in a moist chamber for 15 minutes to allow the platelets to settle into the same focal plane. With the compound microscope, platelets will appear as small, refractile bodies of varying shapes. Platelets in the entire super square should be counted and the platelet number calculated as for manual cell counts. Refer to Chapter 2 for a review of the procedure and calculation. Platelets should number between 150 to 400 $\times$ $10^3/\mu l$.

Bleeding time tests

Bleeding time tests measure the time required for a small controlled wound to stop bleeding and are used to evaluate vascular integrity as well as platelet function. A number of techniques have been developed which are inexpensive and simple to perform. These methods are somewhat imprecise in that they are difficult to standardize. The most commonly used methods in veterinary clinical practice are the buccal bleeding time and cuticle bleeding time tests.

The buccal bleeding time test requires that the animal be placed in lateral recumbency. The upper lip is gently tied back to expose the mucosal surface. A small incision is made in the mucosa at the level of the canine tooth utilizing a disposable capillary lancet. The timer is activated at the time the incision is made. Every 30 seconds thereafter, a dry filter paper is touched to the drop of blood, taking care not to disturb the incision site. The endpoint is noted when the filter paper comes up dry (i.e., incision ceases to bleed freely). In domestic animals, the normal bleeding time is one to five minutes. Cuticle bleeding time tests are also commonly performed on dogs. It is recommended that the dog be anesthetized and placed in lateral recumbency. A toenail is swabbed clean with alcohol and the alcohol allowed to dry before proceeding with the test. A guillotine type clipper is used to clip the apex of the nail and the nail is allowed to bleed freely and undisturbed. The endpoint is noted when bleeding stops. Cuticle bleeding time in dogs ranges from 3 to 9 minutes.

Coagulation time tests

Several types of whole blood clotting time tests are commonly performed in veterinary practice. These are all in vitro methods which evaluate only the intrinsic and common pathways.

The Lee White coagulation time method requires three 13 $\times$ 75 mm tubes which have been warmed in a 37°C water bath or heat block. Three milliliters of blood are collected by venipuncture, and a timer is started at the first appearance of blood in the syringe. One milliliter is immediately placed in each of the three tubes. At 30 second intervals, one of the tubes is tilted and observed for evidence of clot formation. When this tube has clotted, the second and then the third tubes are observed in the same manner. The endpoint is reached when a clot forms in the third tube.

The capillary coagulation time method is performed by making a superficial wound in a peripheral capillary bed. A sterile disposable lancet is used and the timer activated as soon as the incision is made. The first drop of blood is contaminated with tissue fluid and must be wiped away before blood collection. Blood is collected directly into two or three capillary tubes. A small break is made in a tube about every 30 seconds. The endpoint is reached when strands of fibrin can be seen extending over the gap between the two broken ends of the tube.

The activated clotting time test (ACT) is more accurate and precise and takes less time to perform than the previous methods. The Vacutainer system is used and two blood tubes are required. One tube is plain and the second contains diatomaceous earth (DE) which serves to activate the intrinsic pathway. Venipuncture is performed and the plain tube is used to collect the first few drops of blood, which are discarded. The DE tube is then introduced and the timer is activated with the first appearance of blood in this tube. Approximately 2 ml of blood should be collected and the tube gently inverted to mix the blood and DE. The tube is placed immediately in a 37°C heat block. After 30 seconds, the tube is tilted to check for clot formation and then returned to the heat block. The tube should be rechecked every 5 seconds until the blood clots. Normal ACT time for the dog is 60 to 110 seconds and 50 to 75 seconds for the cat. Abnormally prolonged coagulation times are seen in a number of hemostatic defects, such as factor I deficiency and vonWillebrand's disease. Additional testing would be required to determine the specific cause of any abnormality identified with the coagulation time test.

Clot retraction test

The clot retraction test is a simple inexpensive way to evaluate platelet number and function, as well as the intrinsic and common pathways. Blood is drawn into a plain sterile tube and placed in a 37°C water bath or heat block. The tube is examined after 60 minutes for evidence of clot formation and then reexamined periodically for 24 hours. The clot should be retracted in about 4 hours and will appear as a diffuse red mass surrounded by serum. At 24 hours, the clot should be markedly compacted.

Clot retraction is impaired in factor I deficiencies, thrombocytopenia, and other conditions which result in abnormal platelet function. Some coagulation defects may result in complete dissolution of the clot during the 24 hour incubation. Clot retraction may also be abnormal in anemia and polycythemia.

Prothrombin time test

The one-stage prothrombin time (PT) test is used to evaluate the extrinsic coagulation pathway. A plasma sample, collected with a sodium citrate or oxalate anticoagulant, is required. A reagent containing a tissue thromboplastin, usually harvested from rabbit brain tissue, is added to the sample. The test system is then recalcified and the timer activated. The test must be performed at 37°C. The normal time required for clot formation in domestic animals ranges from 6 to 20 seconds. The PT test is most reliable when an instrument such as the fibrometer is used to detect clot formation (Fig. 4-3). A control should also be assayed along with the patient sample.

Activated partial thromboplastin time (APTT)

Defects in the intrinsic coagulation pathway are determined with the APTT test. A citrated plasma sample is required. Two separate reagents are also needed: one containing calcium chloride, and a second which contains an artificially activated thromboplastin and platelet phospholipids. The reagents, patient plasma sample, and a plasma sample from a normal control animal are incubated in a 37°C water bath or heat block for several minutes prior to testing. The thromboplastin reagent and the plasma sample are combined in the heat block. The calcium chloride reagent is then added and the timer activated. Clot formation is evi-

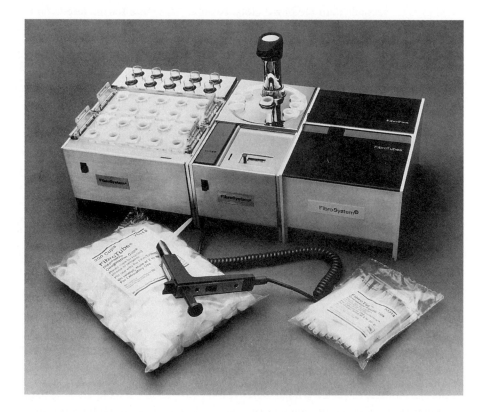

Fig. 4-3. The Fibrometer provides verification of clot formation for coagulation studies. (Photo courtesy Becton-Dickinson/Microbiology Systems.)

dent as a mesh of fibrin strands, visible as a semisolid gel. Automated methods are also available which add reagents in sequence and detect clot formation with an optical beam or electrical current. The specific details of a procedure will vary depending on the manufacturer of the chosen reagents or the instrument. Regardless of the method chosen, results must be obtained in duplicate and then averaged. This average is then compared to the normal control sample which is assayed in the same manner as the patient sample. An APTT result which is 30% greater than the normal control is considered an abnormal finding. APTT times of 12 to 25 seconds are common for domestic animals.

Partial thromboplastin time

The intrinsic coagulation pathway may also be evaluated with the partial thromboplastin time (PTT) test. The methodology for PTT is similar to the APTT, except that the thromboplastin reagent is not in an activated form and therefore normal PTT test time is slightly higher than for the APTT test.

Fibrinogen assay

Several methods are available which can evaluate fibrinogen concentration in a sample. The simplest of these involves filling two microhematocrit tubes with EDTA-treated whole blood. The tubes are centrifuged as for a mHct determination. Plasma protein concentration is measured in one of the tubes, usually with a refractometer. The second tube is then heated for 3 minutes at 56°C, recentrifuged, and the plasma protein concentration determined. Heating causes the precipitation of fibrinogen in the sample. The difference in plasma protein concentration between the two tubes provides an estimate of the fibrinogen concentration in the sample.

Additional evaluations

A number of additional test methodologies are available for coagulation evaluations. Most of these are not commonly performed in veterinary practice but are available in large reference laboratories. These include tests which measure the specific concentration and functional ability of the various blood coagulation factors.

KEY POINTS

1. Hemostasis refers to the ability of the body to maintain the integrity of the blood vessels and fluid.

2. Blood coagulation involves both a mechanical and a chemical phase and culminates in the formation of a fibrin clot.

3. Mechanical hemostasis involves platelet aggregation and activation.

4. Chemical hemostasis may be triggered through either an extrinsic or intrinsic pathway.

5. The chemical pathways involve a series of stepwise reactions known as the coagulation cascade.

6. Both the extrinsic and intrinsic pathways culminate in the activation of factor X, which triggers the reactions of the common pathway.

7. Coagulation defects may be inherited or acquired.

8. The most common inherited bleeding disorder is vonWillebrand's disease, which is especially common in Doberman Pinschers.

9. Acquired coagulation abnormalities may occur secondary to liver disease, vitamin K deficiency, or ingestion of aspirin.

10. A platelet count less than $100 \times 10^3/\mu l$ is termed thrombocytopenia and may be hereditary or acquired.

11. Laboratory tests of hemostasis are designed to evaluate specific portions of the coagulation pathways.

12. For coagulation studies, the preferred anticoagulants are citrates and oxalates.

13. Thrombocyte counts may be performed on a diluted, EDTA-treated blood sample with a hemocytometer.

14. Platelet function may be evaluated with the clot retraction and bleeding time tests.

REVIEW QUESTIONS

1. Define hemostasis.
2. Which coagulation factor activates the extrinsic pathway?
3. What role do platelets play in blood coagulation?
4. True or False. A bleeding disorder in a young animal is most likely an acquired defect.
5. Animals with vonWillebrand's disease may also have a reduction in factor _____ activity.
6. Inadequate consumption or malabsorption or vitamin K results in deficiencies of factors _____, _____, _____, and _____.
7. Define thrombocytopenia.
8. True or False. Platelet function tests can be performed on a whole blood sample that has been treated with EDTA.

9. The activated clotting time test utilizes the compound _____ as a coagulation activating factor.
10. The instrument used to detect clot formation is the _____.
11. List the tests used to evaluate platelet function.
12. The APTT and PTT tests are designed to evaluate the _____ pathway.
13. The extrinsic pathway is evaluated with the _____ test.

ANSWERS TO REVIEW QUESTIONS

1. Hemostasis is maintenance of the integrity of the blood vessels and fluid.
2. The extrinsic pathway is activated by factor III (tissue thromboplastin).
3. Platelets play a role in mechanically plugging small breaks in small blood vessels and providing an initiating coagulation factor.
4. False. A bleeding disorder in a young animal is most likely an inherited defect.
5. Animals with vonWillebrand's disease may also have a reduction in factor VIII activity.
6. Inadequate consumption or malabsorption of vitamin K results in deficiencies of factors II, VII, IX, and X.
7. Thrombocytopenia refers to platelet counts that are below $100 \times 10^3/\mu l$.
8. False. EDTA inhibits platelet function. Citrate or oxalate anticoagulants should be used for platelet function testing.
9. The activated clotting time test utilizes the compound diatomaceous earth as a coagulation activating factor.
10. The instrument used to detect clot formation is the fibrometer.
11. Clot retraction and bleeding time tests are used to evaluate platelet function.
12. The APTT and PTT tests are designed to evaluate the intrinsic pathway.
13. The extrinsic pathway is evaluated with the prothrombin time test.

SELECTED READING

Cotter SM: *Comparative Transfusion Medicine*. Cleveland, 1993, CRC Press.
Dodds WJ: Hemostasis and coagulation. In: Kaneko, editor: *Clinical Biochemistry of Domestic Animals*, ed 3. New York, 1980, Academic Press.
Pittiglio DH, editor: *Clinical Hematology and Fundamentals of Hemostasis*. Philadelphia, 1987, FA Davis Co.
Coles EH: *Veterinary Clinical Pathology*, ed 4. Philadelphia, 1986, WB Saunders Co.
Benjamin M: *Outline of Veterinary Clinical Pathology*, ed 3. Ames, IA, 1978, Iowa State University Press.
Feldman BF: *Hemostasis. The Veterinary Clinics of North America, Small Animal Practice*, vol 18. Philadelphia, 1988, WB Saunders Co.

The immune system

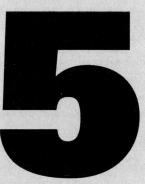

PERFORMANCE OBJECTIVES
After completion of this chapter, the student will:

List the components of the nonadaptive defenses of an organism.

Describe the maturation of the blood lymphocytes.

List the subpopulations of lymphocytes and describe the role of each.

Describe the structure of the immunoglobulins and the role of each in immunity.

List and describe the types of
antigen-antibody reactions that can occur in an organism.

List the parameters to consider in choosing an immunologic test kit.

Differentiate between sensitivity and specificity.

List the methods available for measuring the immune response.

Describe the principle behind the ELISA technique for immunologic testing.

List the general procedure for Coombs testing.

Describe the procedure for cross-matching of blood.

The organs, systems, and specialized cells which are involved in the defense mechanisms of the body are collectively referred to as the immune system. Any substance which is capable of eliciting a response from the immune system is called an antigen. Antigens include substances such as bacteria, viruses, parasites, and similar substances which the immune system can recognize as "foreign." A key factor in this recognition is the ability of certain cells of the immune system to identify molecules on the surface of the antigen which are different from molecules found on the body's own cells. The specific surface marker portion of the substance can therefore be antigenic on its own.

This antigen recognition will frequently result in the formation of specific antibody to neutralize or destroy the antigen. The antibody produced in response to a specific antigen is specific for the surface molecules of that particular antigen. Formation of specific antibody is a function of the adaptive component of the immune system. Adaptive immunity also includes the ability to react and respond quickly to subsequent attacks by the same antigen. This 'memory' ability distinguishes the adaptive and nonadaptive components of the immune system.

Nonadaptive immunity

Nonadaptive defenses provide physical and/or chemical barriers to antigen attack. These are nonspecific defenses in that they do not require recognition of specific surface markers in order to function. They do not require production of antibody and are not capable of 'memory' in subsequent attacks by the same antigen. Nonadaptive defenses generally react and respond in the same manner regardless of the type of antigen involved.

Intact skin and mucous membranes are examples of physical barriers in the nonadaptive immune system. Certain body fluids, such as tears, contain lysozymes which are capable of lysing bacterial cells. Hydrochloric acid, found in the stomach, can also destroy some foreign substances. Certain leukocytes are also involved in nonadaptive defenses. These include specific populations of neutrophils which reside in the respiratory, digestive, and urinary tracts. Resident neutrophils act as scavengers and can phagocytize most infectious agents. Other leukoctyes can initiate an inflammatory response to tissue damage by an invading antigen.

Natural killer (NK) cells also function in nonadaptive defenses. Although the exact lineage of these cells is unknown, NK cells can be found in circulation. These cells appear to be derived from large granular lymphocytes and are capable of direct lysis of infectious agents as well as tumor cells.

Adaptive immunity

In addition to their role in nonadaptive immunity, the blood leukocytes are an integral component of the adaptive immune system. Phagocytic cells such as neutrophils and macrophages must process and present an antigen to specific populations of lymphocytes before antibody can be produced. Other specialized cells in the lymph nodes are also capable of antigen presentation.

Two specific subpopulations of lymphoctyes are responsible for the activities of the immune system. The T-lymphocytes are those that are matured in the thymus. B-lymphocytes mature independent of the thymus in various lymphoid tissues. Morphologically, it is impossible to distinguish these two cell types. Special staining techniques which identify specific surface molecules of these cells must be used for identification.

B-lymphocytes are primarily involved with synthesizing and secreting antibody. During maturation, a B-cell is exposed to antigen by an antigen-presenting cell (APC) and becomes specialized to produce only the antibody which is capable of binding to that specific antigen. Similarly, other groups of B-cells are presented with antigen and mature with the ability to synthesize only that specific antibody. In future attacks by an antigen, only those B-cells which have been previously exposed to the same antigen will be activated and respond with antibody production. Although B-cells can be activated independent of T-cells, interactions with T-cells and substances known as cytokines result in full B-cell activation. Cytokines act as chemical messengers and are produced by B- and T-lymphocytes, monocytes, and macrophages. Interactions of these cells and substances will trigger proliferation of the specific population of B-cells which are capable of producing the necessary antibody. These cells will differentiate into plasma cells and begin to produce and secrete antibody. This is referred to as humoral immunity since the antibody is secreted into the body's fluids or humors. In contrast to humoral immunity, in which the B-cell does not act directly on the antigen, T-lymphocytes are primarily involved in cellular immunity and are capable of direct attacks on an antigen.

T-lymphocytes perform numerous functions in the immune system. As with B-cell activation, antigen must be presented to the appropriate memory T-cell. This sensitized T-cell then enlarges and divides, which activates a group of related T-cells. T-helper cells interact with and help activate B-cells, as well as other cytotoxic cells. Cytotoxic T-cells, also known as killer cells, are granular T-cells which are capable of binding and destroying foreign cells and virally infected cells. Another subset of T-lymphocytes are the T-suppressor cells which help regulate the immune response by inhibiting the activity of cytotoxic cells. The chief mechanisms by which T-cells work is the production and secretion of lymphokines such as interferon and several classes of interleukins. Lymphokines are simply cytokines which are produced by lymphocytes. These substances each have specific target cells and result in the activation of many cells in the immune system. Another cytokine, tumor necrosis factor (TNF), is also produced by T-cells. TNF can destroy tumor cells and is also capable of attacking some viruses and parasites.

The mechanisms by which an animal produces antibody are utilized in vaccination of animals against disease. A vaccine contains an inactive form of an antigen which is not capable of causing disease but contains the specific surface markers which the body can identify as foreign. This results in antibody production similar to that which would occur in a natural infection. Should the animal be subsequently exposed to the antigen, specific antibody will already be available to act against the disease agent. An overview of the immune response is found in Fig. 5-1.

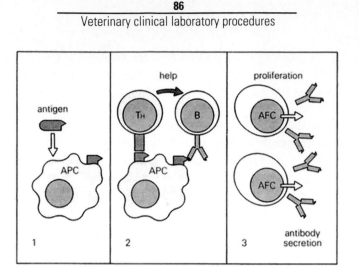

Fig. 5-1. Overview of the immune response. (From Roitt I, Brostoff J, Male D: *Immunology*, ed. 3, London, 1993, Mosby–Year Book Europe.)

Antibody structure

Antibodies are soluble globular proteins collectively referred to as immunoglobulins (Igs). They are symmetrical molecules with monomers that consist of two pairs of polypeptide chains. One of the pairs comprises the constant region, also referred to as the Fc region. This site is capable of binding to receptors on several types of body cells, such as T-cells and macrophages. The polypeptide chains of the constant region are similar within each of the Ig classes. The second pair of polypeptide chains comprises the variable region. This is the region which interacts with and binds to specific antigen. Immunoglobulins are unique for each antigen, with the variable region closely matched to the surface markers on the antigen which triggered the antibody production. Each Ig monomer is bivalent; that is, it contains two identical antigen-binding sites. The variable portion is also referred to as fragment of antigen binding (Fab). Five distinct classes of immunoglobulins are produced by B-cells—IgG, IgM, IgE, IgD, and IgA (Fig. 5-2).

The most abundant circulating immunoglobulin is IgG. It comprises approximately 75% of circulating Ig and remains in circulation longest. IgG is a relatively small monomer which is capable of entering tissue spaces and is usually produced during a secondary immune response. The first antibody type produced in response to an antigen is IgM. IgM is a pentameric molecule (i.e., contains 5 monomers) and comprises about 5% of circulating Ig. IgM is relatively large and is therefore unable to enter tissue spaces. IgE is usually present in very small amounts and is similar in structure to IgG. Increased levels of IgE are seen during hypersensitivity reactions. IgE also plays a crucial role in the immune response to parasitic worm infections. IgA comprises about 20% of circulating antibody and both monomeric and dimeric forms exist. IgA is primarily involved with protecting body sur-

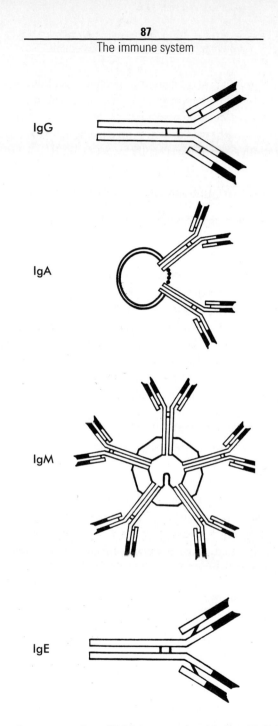

Fig. 5-2. Schematic representation of IgM (pentamer) and IgG and IgE (monomers) and IgA (dimer). (From Gershwin: *Immunology and Immunopathology of Domestic Animals*, ed. 2, St. Louis, 1995, Mosby.)

faces that are in contact with the external environment. Concentrations of IgA can be found associated with intestinal mucosa and respiratory passages and in body secretions such as tears and saliva. IgD has not been demonstrated to exist in all animals. It is a monomer which, when present, is in very low abundance. Its exact function is not completely known, but it may be involved with activation of B-cells by acting on B-cell antigen receptors.

Antigen-antibody interactions

The specific type of reaction that occurs between an antigen and a specific antibody depends upon the nature of the antigen as well as the class of Ig which responds. Some of these reactions also require components of the complement system. The complement system consists of a series of soluble proteins which are involved in certain antigen-antibody interactions. This system is discussed further in the next section of this chapter.

Precipitation reactions involve either very small, soluble, particulate antigens or soluble molecular antigenic material (e.g., bacterial endotoxins). The combination of the antigen with specific antibody (usually IgG) forms an insoluble complex. This precipitate may form on cell surfaces and is then removed either by a phagocytic cell or via some excretory process. In some cases, the precipitant itself causes pathology. For example, precipitation of bacterial fragments in the glomerular membrane elicits an inflammatory response and can result in glomerular nephritis.

Neutralization reactions involve either large molecular antigens or very small particulate material (e.g., viruses). Specific antibody, usually IgA or IgG, coats the antigen and thus inhibits its activity. The antibody-coated antigen can then be more easily phagocytized.

Lytic reactions between cellular antigens and IgM or IgA result in the formation of small pores on the surface membrane of the antigen. Activated complement then interacts and the resulting disruption of the osmotic balance within the cell causes lysis of the antigen.

Opsonization reactions are rare in vivo but are sometimes used for in vitro testing of the immune system. Large particulate antigens are cross-linked with antibody, forming large insoluble complexes.

The complement system

The series of 25 soluble chemicals which function in humoral immunity are collectively referred to as complement. The complement system can be activated through one of two pathways. Once activated, a series of chemical reactions, known as the complement cascade, occurs which can result in lysis of the antigen or enhanced phagocytosis (Fig. 5-3). The components of the complement system are numbered C1 through C9, with some having several subunits designated with letters.

The classical pathway is activated when C1 is bound to an antigen-antibody complex. In the presence of calcium, this catalyzes a series of reactions of other complement mole-

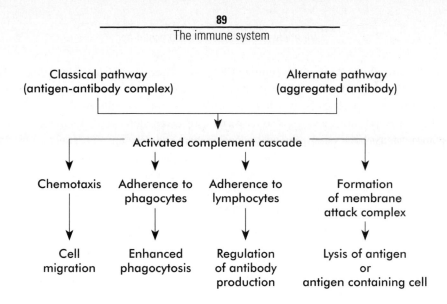

Fig. 5-3. Effects of complement activation.

cules which have numerous physiologic effects. The activated components of complement act as chemotactic factors which attract and activate neutrophils and other granulocytes. Phagocytosis is enhanced when complement is bound to an antigen-antibody complex. In addition, the completion of the complement cascade results in cell lysis by the formation of a membrane attack complex on the surface of the antigen or antigen-containing cell. The alternate pathway of complement activation can be triggered by the presence of large amounts of antigenic material such as viral capsular material and bacterial endotoxins. Large aggregations of antibody will also activate the cascade. The alternate pathway is especially important in young animals whose immune systems are immature, since it does not require the production of specific antibody.

Immunologic defects

Disorders of the immune system are often related to production of excess immunoglobulin (hypergammaglobulinemia) or inability to produce an adequate amount of immunoglobulin (hypogammaglobulinemia). These defects are usually acquired secondarily to some other disease. Tumors of lymphoid tissues may result in uncontrolled proliferation of lympho-cytes and subsequent hypergammaglobulinemia. Viruses, such as canine distemper, par-vovirus, and feline leukemia virus, can compromise the function of various components of the immune system. Functional Ig defects include allergies and anaphylactic reactions.

Allergic reactions result from interaction of mast cells and antigen. IgE, produced as a result of a prior exposure to an antigen, can be found attached to mast cells. On secondary exposure, this surface IgE will bind the antigen. If two such IgE molecules bind the same antigen, the cross-linking will cause the mast cell to degranulate. Mast cell granules contain vasoactive substances, such as histamine. These substances have many physiologic effects, including dilation of blood vessels, chemotaxis of eosinophils, and contraction of smooth muscle. It is these specific effects which cause the symptoms of allergy.

Rapid absorption of a large amount of antigen can result in an anaphylactic reaction. The animal must have been previously sensitized to the antigen. Subsequent exposure to large amounts of the antigen can result in generalized mast cell degranulation. The sudden release of these large amounts of vasoactive substances may cause anaphylactic shock and the animal may die.

MEASURING IMMUNE RESPONSE

Serologic tests which demonstrate the activity of the immune system are a vital tool in veterinary practice. Breakthroughs in immunologic research have refined the methods and reagents used in these tests. The primary tool which led to these improvement is the monoclonal antibody technique. This has allowed for the large-scale production of antibody capable of reacting with a variety of antigenic materials.

Methods of measuring the immune system are primarily designed to demonstrate the presence of either an antigen or a specific antibody in a sample. The majority of these tests require a serum sample. The immune reaction is then carried out in vitro with the addition of a substance to make the results visible. Most serologic tests are only qualitative and do not provide information regarding the amount of antigen or antibody that is present in a sample.

Choosing the correct type of test kit is a crucial decision for the smooth functioning of the laboratory. The technician must be familiar with the various methodologies employed as well as the sensitivity and specificity of each type. Sensitivity refers to the ability of the test to identify all animals that are truly positive for a given reaction procedure. A large number of false negative results indicates a test with low sensitivity. Specificity is a measure of the numbers of false positive results which a test produces. No test can provide both 100% sensitivity and 100% specificity. The cost of a particular test is also a consideration, as well as the ease and speed at which it can be performed. Many tests provide a means to batch samples. The technician can run multiple samples within the same test format at the same time. This saves both time and money as only one set of controls needs to be run for each batch. Some test kits are provided as stat tests; that is, they are designed to run only one sample at a time. These tests are generally easier to run but tend to be more costly and frequently do not have true positive and negative controls.

Quality control for immunologic testing is vital to ensuring accuracy of results. Most test kits are supplied with two separate control sera vials. One vial is the negative control and the other contains a substance (either antigen or antibody) which will react positively in the test system. When these controls react appropriately, the technician can verify that the results for the patient sample are accurate. Comparing the test results for both the positive and negative control sera can help to differentiate weak positive results from errors in testing which cause false positive results.

Precipitation methods

Immunodiffusion is a widely used type of test which is usually carried out in an agar plate. A central well is cut into the agar and several additional wells are cut around the circumference. An antigen is placed in the central well. Several additional wells are filled with test sample (patient serum) and others with known positive control serum. The reagents diffuse toward one another in the agar gel. A precipitate forms at the point where diffusing antigen and diffusing antibody meet. If no antibody was present in the test sample, no precipitation will be found between the sample well and the central well. This test can also be carried out utilizing a central well of purified antibody to detect the presence of specific antigen in a sample. The Coggin's test for equine infectious anemia uses this methodology.

Radialimmunodiffusion is a precipitation reaction that can be used to quantitate the amount of a specific antigen in a sample. Specific antibody is incorporated into the agar and patient sample is added to wells cut into the agar. As the patient serum diffuses into the agar, a circular area of precipitation forms around those wells containing the antigen. The radius of the circle is measured and compared with the size of a precipitate circle for a known concentration of antigen.

Immunoelectrophoresis is an additional type of precipitation test. A serum sample is added to a plate which has been coated with agar gel. The plate is then exposed to an electric current which causes the proteins in the sample to migrate through the gel. Each protein will migrate a specific distance based on variations in their surface charges and molecular weight as well as the pH and voltage of the test system. Dye can be added to the system to identify and quantitate each separate component. Another variation of the technique incorporates antigen into grooves in the gel. As the proteins migrate and antigen diffuses, bands of precipitation form with the corresponding specific immunoglobulins. The length of the precipitin band corresponds to the amount of antibody present.

Agglutination tests

Antibodies to large, particulate antigens can be easily detected with an agglutination test. The addition of specific antigen to samples containing such antibodies will result in cross-linking of the antigen and antibody and the formation of large, insoluble complexes which are readily visible. Agglutination can also be induced with antibodies to small, soluble antigens by attaching them to another particle (e.g., latex beads). The antigen-bead complex is then added to the patient serum sample. If the sample contains specific antibody, agglutination will be visible. Either of the above types of agglutination reactions can also be used to detect specific antigen in a sample. In veterinary practice, agglutination tests are used to detect and diagnose brucellosis and toxoplasmosis (Fig. 5-4).

A similar methodology is used to detect and quantitate antigens which are nonagglutinating. Specific antibody is incubated with the patient serum sample. Purified antigen-coated latex beads are then added to the test system. If the patient sample contained the specific antigen, the addition of antibody will form antigen-antibody complexes. The antigen-bead complexes added subsequently will not agglutinate since antibody has already complexed with antigen in the patient serum. This type of test is referred to as an agglutination inhibition. A positive agglutination inhibition assay indicates the presence of antigen in the patient sample and is nonagglutinating. This type of test can be applied to quantitate substances such as enzymes and hormones by using serial dilutions of specific antibody.

ELISA testing

The majority of commercially available serology kits for veterinary practice utilize the technique known as enzyme-linked immunosorbent assay (ELISA). The test can be designed to detect either the presence of an antigen or a specific antibody. Several test formats are available which utilize the ELISA methodology. The most common type is the microwell test. For detection of a particular antigen in a sample, microwells are manufactured to contain a specific antibody attached to the wall of the well. These wells are supplied as a component of test kits which also contain all needed reagents to carry out the assay. Microwell tests also contain reagent bottles of positive and negative control material. The patient sample is added to the well. If the specific antigen is present in the sample, it will become attached to the specific antibody on the surface of the well. An enzyme-linked antibody is then added to the test system. If antigen has bound previously, the enzyme-linked antibody will attach to that complex. Subsequent addition of a chromogenic substrate for the enzyme allows positive visualization that the reaction has occurred (Fig. 5-5). ELISA tests for specific antibody are similar to those described above, except that antigen is attached to the well surface. If present in the patient sample, specific antibody will attach to this antigen. Subsequent addition of an enzyme-linked anti-antibody and substrate will make the reaction visible.

Microwell ELISA tests tend to be less expensive and more accurate than other test methodologies (Fig. 5-6). Filter ELISA kits have become popular due to their ease of operation. Many of these filter tests, however, do not contain true positive and negative controls. Instead, procedural controls are incorporated into the devices which verify only that all reagents have been properly added to the system.

Radioimmunoassay

Radioimmunoassay testing is done primarily in research laboratories. The test principle is similar to the ELISA technique, except that a radioisotope is used in place of the enzyme. The amount of either antigen or antibody in the patient sample can then be quantified by measuring the level of radioactivity remaining in the wells after the reaction has taken place.

Fluorescent antibody (FA) testing

Although not commonly performed in veterinary practice, fluorescent testing is available at most veterinary reference laboratories. These test procedures are frequently used to verify a

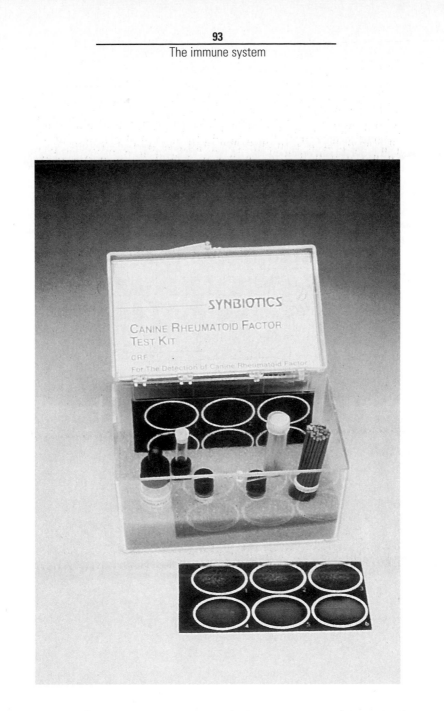

Fig. 5-4. An example of an agglutination test kit. (Photo courtesy of Synbiotics Corp.)

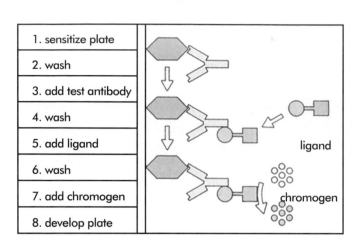

| 1. sensitize plate |
| 2. wash |
| 3. add test antibody |
| 4. wash |
| 5. add ligand |
| 6. wash |
| 7. add chromogen |
| 8. develop plate |

Fig. 5-5. Principle of ELISA reaction. (From Roitt I, Brostoff J, Male D: *Immunology*, ed. 3, London, 1993, Mosby–Year Book Europe.)

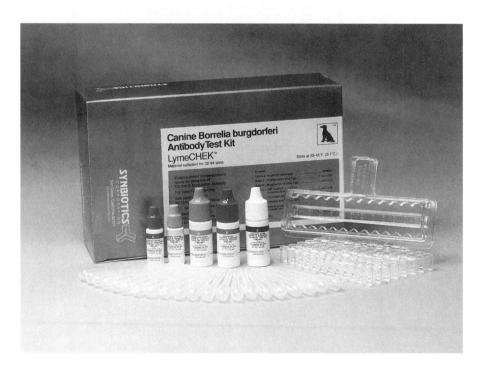

Fig. 5-6. ELISA Test Kits for Canine *B. burgdorferi*. (Photo courtesy of Synbiotics Corp.)

tentative diagnosis made by the veterinarian. Two methodologies are available, both of which detect the presence of specific antibody in a sample (Fig. 5-7). Direct fluorescent testing techniques are most often used for bacterial antigens. Patient sample is added to a test slide which has been precoated with a dye-conjugated antigen. The dye combines with specific antibody, if present in the patient sample. The slide is then examined using a special microscope designed for fluorescent microscopy. For cellular antigens, the cell will appear outlined with fluorescent material.

Indirect fluorescent antibody (IFA) techniques are more commonly employed than direct techniques and are especially useful in detecting antibody to viral agents. Patient sample is incubated on a slide which contains the specific test antigen. The slide is then washed to remove any unbound antibody. Fluorescent-labelled anti-antibody is added to the system. The slide is then examined microscopically. Any fluorescence indicates a positive test result.

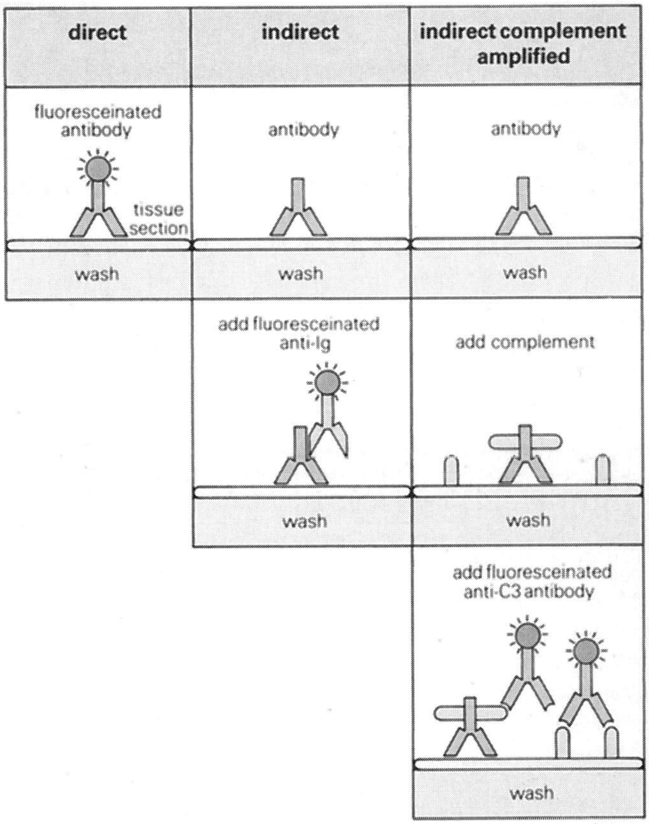

direct	indirect	indirect complement amplified
fluoresceinated antibody · tissue section	antibody	antibody
wash	wash	wash
	add fluoresceinated anti-Ig	add complement
	wash	wash
		add fluoresceinated anti-C3 antibody
		wash

Fig. 5-7. Fluorescent antibody technique. (From Roitt I, Brostoff J, Male D: *Immunology*, ed. 3, London, 1993, Mosby–Year Book Europe.)

Coombs testing

The presence of inappropriate antibodies (i.e., antibodies against the body's own tissues) are detected with the Coombs test (Fig. 5-8). The Direct Coombs reaction is used to detect antibody which has attacked the body's own erythrocytes. Indirect Coombs testing detects circulating self-antibody.

A positive Direct Coombs test provides evidence of hemolytic disease. The procedure involves incubating the suspect sample with an antigammaglobulin which can react against that species' immunoglobulins. If the erythrocytes in the sample are coated with self-antibody, the reaction will result in visible hemagglutination. A positive indirect Coombs test indicates the presence of circulating antibodies against the body's own tissues. In order to visualize the reaction, patient sample is incubated with erythrocytes from a normal animal. If antibody is present in the patient sample, it will bind these erythrocytes. Subsequent addition of an antigammaglobulin for the species being tested will result in hemagglutination.

Antibody titers

Although not routinely performed in the veterinary practice laboratory, antibody titer tests are frequently needed by the clinician to distinguish between active infection and prior exposure to certain antigens. This is particularly important when there is no reliable antigen test available. Titer refers to the greatest dilution at which a patient sample no longer yields a positive result for presence of a specific antibody. The test requires making serial dilutions of a sample. Each dilution is then examined for the presence of the antibody. The reciprocal of the greatest dilution which still elicits a positive test result is the titer. A high titer often indicates active infection. Low titers usually indicate previous exposure to the specific antigen.

Blood groups and immunity

Under certain conditions, the surface marker molecules on erythrocytes can be antigenic. The specific markers present in an individual animal are genetically determined and are referred to as blood group antigens. The number of blood groups is variable among species. In the equine and canine, there are at least eight identifiable blood groups. Cats have three identifiable blood group types.

Transfusion reactions can occur if an animal is given blood which contains cell surface antigens that are different from the animal's own erythrocytes. The presence of this foreign antigen often results in the production of antibody to those specific surface markers on the transfused cell membrane. Subsequent transfusion of the same blood group type will then result in agglutination of the transfused cells due to the attachment of the antibodies to the cell surface.

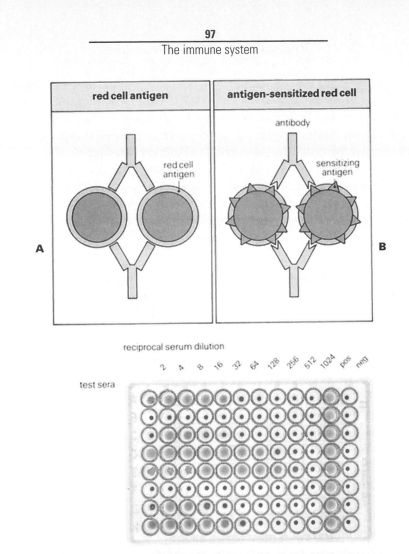

Fig. 5-8. Principles of the Coombs reaction, **A**, direct Coombs test; **B**, indirect Coombs test. (From Roitt I, Brostoff J, Male D: *Immunology*, ed. 3, London, 1993, Mosby–Year Book Europe.)

Canine blood groups are designated as DEA-1.1, DEA-1.2, DEA-3, DEA-4, DEA-5, DEA-6, DEA-7, and DEA-8. DEA-7 is actually not a true erythrocyte antigen, but is adsorbed to the red blood cell membrane from the plasma. About 70% of dogs are negative for this antigen and have naturally occuring DEA-7 antibodies. Should a DEA-7 negative dog be given DEA-7 positive blood, a transfusion reaction is likely. DEA-1.1 and 1.2 negative dogs do not have naturally occurring DEA-1 antibody but will produce this antibody if transfused with DEA positive blood. Subsequent administration of DEA-1 positive blood will cause a transfusion reaction. With the remaining canine blood types, transfusion reactions do not seem to result when transfused blood is mismatched.

Cats have only three blood groups, designated A, B, or AB. Cats with blood type B have strong, naturally occuring antibodies to type A. Transfusion reactions are severe when type A blood is given to type B cats. When type B blood is given to a type A cat, transfusion reaction is less likely, but the life cycle of the transfused erythrocytes is greatly reduced as compared with the life span expected of properly matched blood.

Eight blood groups are recognized in the equine. These are designated A, C, D, K, P, Q, T, and U. Since each of these blood groups has multiple alleles, the probability of any two individual animals having the same blood type is quite small. Cattle have eleven blood group systems and sheep have seven. As with the horse, each group has multiple alleles. In these species, blood group types can be used to verify the parentage of a particular animal.

Typing and cross-matching of blood

Determination of blood type requires the use of antisera which consist of antibodies specific for each possible blood type of a given species. Commercial antisera for canine and feline group testing have recently become available. The procedure requires a whole blood sample collected with EDTA, heparin, or acid-citrate-dextrose (ACD) anticoagulant. The blood is centrifuged at 1000 G for 10 minutes. After removal of the plasma and buffy coat, the erythrocytes are washed three times in a saline solution and resuspended. The red cell suspension is distributed among as many tubes as required for the number of blood type antisera being tested. A small amount (usually 0.1 ml) of the antisera in question is added to the appropriately labeled tube. The tubes are incubated for 15 minutes at room temperature and then recentrifuged for fifteen seconds at 1000 G. Each tube is examined for evidence of hemolysis or agglutination, both microscopically and macroscopically. Weak positive results may require additional testing.

Blood typing of large animals is impractical for routine analysis prior to transfusion. Literally thousands of different antisera would be required due to the large number of different blood groups possible in the sheep, cow, and horse.

In the absence of commercial antisera, cross-matching of a blood donor and recipient animals will reduce the possibility of transfusion reaction. The procedure for cross-matching requires both a serum and a whole blood sample and is divided into two parts. Red cell suspensions, collected as for the blood typing procedure, are prepared. The Major Cross Match procedure involves the addition of a few drops of serum from the recipient animal to a few drops of washed cells from the donor. The mixture is incubated and then centrifuged. The presence of hemolysis or agglutination, either micro- or macroscopically, would indicate a blood type mismatch. The Minor Cross Match procedure is similar, except that donor serum and recipient cells are used. Both of these procedures should be performed on all animals with unknown blood types that require transfusion. Two controls are utilized for the test which consist of running the procedure using donor cells together with donor serum and recipient cells together with recipient serum.

KEY POINTS

1. Antigens are substances viewed as foreign by the body.

2. The ability of the immune system to recognize an antigen depends on the specific surface markers of the antigen.

3. The immune system consists of both an adaptive and nonadaptive component.

4. Nonadaptive immunity involves physical barriers, chemical lytic agents, and phagocytic cells.

5. T-lymphocytes are matured in the thymus and are primarily involved in the production of cytokines.

6. B-lymphocytes mature independent of the thymus and are primarily involved in the production of antibody.

7. Cytokines are chemical messengers produced by a variety of cells which interact with components of the immune system.

8. Five classes of immunoglobulins are produced by B-cells. Each class has a specific role in immunity.

9. The complement system is a series of chemicals which interact with the cells of the immune system.

10. Serologic tests are designed to identify the presence or absence of an antigen or specific antibody.

11. Most commercially available tests for measuring the immune response utilize the ELISA technology.

12. Transfusion of foreign cells can result in antibody production and transfusion reaction.

13. Cross-matching of donor and recipient blood is essential to minimizing the possibility of transfusion reaction.

REVIEW QUESTIONS

1. List the components of the nonadaptive immune system.
2. What is the role of cytokines in immunity?
3. Secretion of antibody is performed by _____ and is referred to as _____ immunity.
4. List the subpopulations of T-lymphocytes.
5. Describe the general structure of immunoglobulins.
6. List the classes of immunoglobulins.
7. Which Ig class is involved in hypersensitivity reactions?
8. What is complement and what role does it play in immunity?
9. What factors should be considered when choosing a serologic test kit?
10. Describe the principle behind the ELISA test for specific antigen.
11. Define titer.
12. Describe the general procedure for cross-matching of blood.

Veterinary clinical laboratory procedures

ANSWERS TO REVIEW QUESTIONS

1. The nonadaptive immune system consists of physical barriers, such as skin and mucous membrane, chemical agents, such as those found in saliva and tears, and phagocytic cells that reside in tissues.
2. Cytokines are chemical messengers that stimulate cells of the immune system.
3. Secretion of antibody is performed by B-lymphocytes and is referred to as humoral immunity.
4. Subpopulations of T-lymphocytes include helper T-cells, cytotoxic T-cells, and suppressor T-cells.
5. Immunoglobulins are symmetrical globular protein molecules composed of two pairs of polypeptide chains. One pair makes up the constant region; the second pair makes up the variable region, which is the site of antigen binding.
6. The classes of immunoglobulins are IgG, IgM, IgA, IgE, and IgD.
7. IgE is involved in hypersensitivity reactions.
8. Complement is a series of soluble proteins which interact with components of the immune system and increase the efficiency of the activity of those components.
9. When choosing a serologic test kit, the test sensitivity and specificity should be considered, as well as the cost and ease of operation.
10. The ELISA test for specific antigen utilizes a specific antibody which is bound to either a well or membrane. When an antigen-containing sample is added, the antigen will bind this antibody. A second antibody enzyme-linked antibody with chromogen is added to visualize the reaction.
11. Titer is the greatest dilution at which a sample no longer yields a positive result for the presence of specific antibody or antigen.
12. Red cell suspensions are prepared.
    Major Cross Match—add a few drops of serum from the recipient animal to a few drops of washed cells from the donor. Incubate and then centrifuge. Examine micro- and macroscopically for hemolysis or agglutination. Minor Cross Match—same as Major cross-match, except that donor serum and recipient cells are used. Controls—run the procedure using donor cells together with donor serum and recipient cells together with recipient serum.

SELECTED READING

Tizard I: *An Introduction to Veterinary Immunology*, ed 2. Philadelphia, 1982, WB Saunders Co.

Roitt IM, Brostoff J, Male DK: *Immunology*, ed 2. St. Louis, 1989, CV Mosby Co.

Abbas AK, Lichtman AH, Pober JS: *Cellular and Molecular Immunology*. Philadelphia, 1991, WB Saunders.

Barrett JT: *Textbook of Immunology: an introduction to immunochemistry and immunobiology*, ed 5. St. Louis, 1988, CV Mosby Co.

Coles EH: *Veterinary Clinical Pathology*, ed 4. Philadelphia, 1986, WB Saunders Co.

National Institutes of Health: *Understanding Immunology*. Pub. No. 90-529. US Dept of Health and Human Services. Public Health Service, Washington D.C., 1990.

Blood chemistry

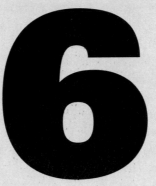

PERFORMANCE OBJECTIVES
After completion of this chapter, the student will:

List the types of instruments used in clinical chemistry testing.

Differentiate between an endpoint and a kinetic assay.

List the chemical tests used to evaluate liver function in an organism.

Describe the common methods for total serum protein measurement.

Explain the dye-binding technique for albumin testing.

Describe the metabolism of bilirubin in the normal animal.

Explain the procedure for the Diazo test for bilirubin.

Describe the procedure for dye clearance test in both large and small animals.

Define "enzyme activity unit" and explain the general principle for enzyme testing.

List the chemical tests used to evaluate kidney function in an organism.

Describe the principle behind the Jaffe reaction for creatinine testing.

Explain the procedure for calculation of the creatinine clearance rate.

List the tests used to evaluate pancreatic function in an organism.

Describe the general principle behind amylase and lipase testing.

Describe the metabolism of glucose in the diabetic individual.

Explain the procedure for the glucose tolerance test.

Explain the procedure for serum calcium analysis.

Describe the principle of direct potentiometric analysis of serum electrolytes.

D eterminations of levels of the various chemical constituents in blood can provide valuable diagnostic information to the clinician. The chemicals being assayed are generally associated with particular organ functions and are of several types. They may be enzymes produced by the organs or metabolites and metabolic by-products which are processed by certain organs. Analysis of these components usually requires a carefully collected blood serum sample. Plasma may be utilized in some cases. Chemical measurements should be completed within one hour after blood collection. If testing is to be delayed, freezing of the sample will preserve the integrity of most constituents. Freezing may interfere with some test methodologies. Certain anticoagulants may also interfere with particular chemical analyses. The technician must be familiar with each test methodology used to avoid errors caused by improper sample collection or handling. Refer to Chapter 2 for a review of sample collection and handling procedures.

As reasonably priced automated chemistry analyzers have become available, more veterinary practices have been able to perform these assays in-house. In-house testing provides results more quickly and at more flexible times than if the tests are performed at a commercial veterinary reference lab and can provide an additional source of income for the busy veterinary practice.

Instruments designed for clinical chemistry analysis employ either photometric or electrochemical principles. In general, photometric procedures involve addition of reagents to a serum sample which causes the sample to develop color. The intensity of that color is directly related to the concentration of the chemical constituent which the reagent acted upon. Electrochemical devices are designed to detect changes in oxidation status as electrons are gained or lost from a test system. Automated electrolyte analyzers and pH meters utilize this technology.

The vast majority of both manual and automated methodologies for clinical chemistry testing utilize photometric instrumentation. One application of the photometric principle is the spectrophotometer. Most in-house chemistry analyzers employ the principles of spectrophotometry. These automated analyzers use either liquid reagents or slides which contain dry reagents (Fig. 6-1). Liquid reagents may be purchased in bulk or in unitized disposable cuvettes. Bulk liquid reagents are least expensive but require additional handling and storage space. Some reagents are flammable and toxic. The purchase of unitized reagents eliminates the potential hazard associated with handling these reagents, but they are more

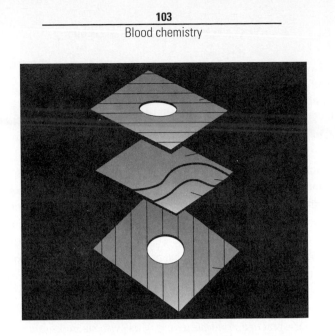

Fig. 6-1. An exploded view of a "dry" reagent clinical chemistry slide. Reagents are located on the central pad of the slide and sample is added to this area. (Reprinted courtesy of Eastman Kodak Co.)

costly. Dry slide reagents pose little, if any, handling or storage hazard and require little storage space, but can be quite expensive.

Regardless of the instrumentation or reagents chosen, a thorough knowledge of anatomy and physiology is essential to the selection of appropriate test methodologies. Methodologies are reviewed by several professional associations to ensure that the methods are valid for measuring the specific chemical constituent in a particular species. Strict adherence to quality control procedures is vital to minimizing any potential sources of error in testing.

Liver function tests

Hepatic cells exhibit extreme diversity of function. As a result, there are over 100 different types of tests to evaluate liver function. Hepatocytes are capable of regeneration if damaged. The rate of regeneration varies with the age of the animal, as well as the nature and extent of the damage. Usually, liver disease is greatly progressed by the time clinical signs appear. The regenerative capabilities of the liver present difficulties in determining the extent of liver damage in disease. Liver function tests are frequently used to establish the rate of progression or regression of liver damage. Serial determinations of certain liver function tests can determine whether liver function is returning to normal or worsening. Liver function tests are designed to measure levels of substances which are produced or modified by the liver or are released when hepatocytes are damaged.

Protein measurements

Many diseases may result in abnormal levels of plasma proteins. Alterations in plasma protein concentrations are frequently seen in certain cases of liver disease and in kidney disease as well. The proteins found in plasma are primarily of two types: (1) albumin, and (2) globulins. The globulin portion includes alpha, beta, and gamma globulins. The globulin constituents represent a variety of molecules and their building blocks, such as hemoglobin, coagulation factors, and immunoglobulins. Albumin is the most abundant protein in serum. Its primary role is in maintenance of the osmotic balance in blood as well as acting as a carrier molecule for other substances, such as bilirubin, hormones, and certain drugs. Direct chemical measurements of globulins are rarely done. Usually, total protein and albumin determinations are made and the difference between these two measurements represents the globulins. Similarly, the concentration of coagulation proteins can be estimated by subtracting the concentration of total protein in serum from that found in the plasma.

Total protein

In the small veterinary practice, total protein is usually measured with a refractometer (see Chapter 1). This instrument gives a measurement of the refractive index of a substance. The proteins represent the major solid component in plasma or serum, and thus the refractive index is a function of the total concentration of protein in the serum.

The majority of chemical analyses to measure total protein utilize the Biuret method. Biuret reagent is composed of copper ions at an alkaline pH. When combined with serum or plasma, the reagent forms a violet-colored complex with molecules which contain three or more peptide bonds. The intensity of the violet color is a function of the number of peptide bonds present and is therefore proportional to the total protein present in the sample. The colored complex has maximum absorbance at 540 nm and can be quantified with a spectrophotometric analysis using either a standard curve or a one point calibration. The Biuret procedure is linear (i.e., adheres to Beer's law) up to about 12 g/dl.

Hyperproteinemia is an abnormal increase in total protein. This is commonly seen in patients that are dehydrated and is in fact not a true increase in protein. With dehydration, the decrease in volume of body fluids creates an artificial increase in the concentration of solid materials in the fluid. Similarly, fluid overload from intravenous therapy will mimic hypoproteinemia (i.e., decrease in total protein). More commonly, hypoproteinemia is the result of decreased production of protein as in advanced stages of chronic liver disease.

Albumin

The most commonly performed technique for albumin testing is the dye-binding method. This test involves conjugating albumin to a biological dye at a specific pH. The resulting colored solution is measured in the spectrophotometer. The dye chosen must be extremely sensitive and not capable of cross-reacting with other protein components in the serum. The principal dye for use in veterinary clinical practice is bromocresol green (BCG). At a pH of 2 to 4, BCG forms a blue-colored complex with albumin. This complex has maximum absorbance at 590 nm. This procedure is linear to 6 g/dl. Care must be taken in sample collection if plasma is used. The use of oxalate anticoagulants can decrease plasma albumin measurements. Heparin may increase albumin readings.

Protein separation techniques

A number of techniques have been developed to separate the various proteins in plasma or serum. These procedures are not commonly performed in veterinary practice but may be done in some reference labs and research facilities.

Protein fractionation involves the use of salt solutions of varying ionic concentrations. Each of the protein components in the serum will precipitate out of the solutions based on differences in their relative solubility in these different ionic solutions. Electrophoresis and chromatography are performed in research facilities. Both techniques require highly specialized and expensive equipment. Centrifugation at high speeds can also separate the various protein fractions in serum. A centrifuge which is capable of maintaining very high G forces for prolonged periods is required.

Bilirubin testing

Bilirubin is an insoluble molecule derived from the breakdown of hemoglobin in the spleen. The molecule is loosely bound to albumin and transported to the liver. Hepatic cells then metabolize and conjugate the bilirubin to glucuronic acid, which increases the solubility of the molecule. Bilirubin glucuronide is secreted from the hepatocytes and becomes a component of bile. Bacteria within the intestinal tract reduce this compound to a group of related compounds which are collectively referred to as urobilinogen. Urobilinogen is then oxidized to urobilin and excreted in feces. A secondary pathway for bilirubin excretion involves the absorption of bilirubin glucuronide or urobilinogen directly into the blood. These compounds are then excreted as urinary bilirubin and urobilinogen via the kidney (Fig. 6-2).

Measurements of the circulating levels of these various populations of bilirubin can help to pinpoint the cause of jaundice, which is an increase in blood bilirubin. In most species, bilirubin glucuronide comprises about one third of circulating levels of bilirubin. Alterations in this ratio can indicate a pathologic condition. The prehepatic bilirubin, bound to albumin, comprises about two thirds of the total. Differences in the relative solubility and reactivity of these populations allow each to be quantified. The reagent used most often for bilirubin testing is the diazo reagent. Diazo reagent is an aqueous solution of sodium nitrite and sulfanilic and hydrochloric acids. Bilirubin glucuronide will react with this reagent immediately and form a colored substance which can be measured in the spectrophotometer. Prehepatic, unconjugated bilirubin is not soluble in diazo reagent and requires the addition of alcohol to react. The addition of an alcohol to the test system gives a measure of the total bilirubin present in the patient sample. The concentration of direct-reacting bilirubin is then subtracted from this total to yield the concentration of indirect-reacting portion. The diazo reagent test is sensitive to about 20 g/dl. As with all photometric analyses, any condition which alters serum color or clarity will introduce error into the test system. Excessively hemolyzed or lipemic samples require the use of a serum blank. Bilirubin is extremely sensitive to ultraviolet light. Bilirubin standards, as well as the

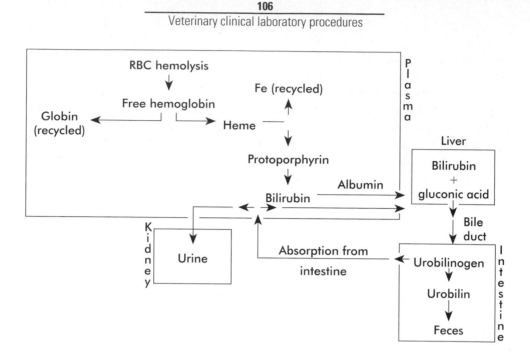

Fig. 6-2. Normal pathway of bilirubin metabolism in the mammal.

patient sample, must be protected from prolonged exposure to UV light.

In most species, an increase in circulating levels of unconjugated bilirubin is seen with a variety of conditions which are characterized by increased erythrocyte destruction. Increases in levels of conjugated bilirubin usually indicate obstructive disease of the bile duct system. Increases in levels of both populations of bilirubin indicate hepatocellular disease. In addition, damaged cells often impair circulation within the liver so that conjugated bilirubin is not released into the bile duct. Interpretation of bilirubin test results is complicated by normal physiologic differences among species. The equine, for example, excretes very little unconjugated bilirubin in health or disease.

Serum bile acids

Bile acids are produced in the liver and secreted into bile by the hepatocytes. These compounds aid in normal digestion of lipids. In normal animals, serum bile acid levels are quite low. In certain disease conditions which alter the circulation within the liver, bile acids will be absorbed into the blood. Tests to measure serum bile acids levels have become readily available only recently. These assays have proved valuable in ruling out extrahepatic disorders and in following the course of hepatic disease. It is crucial that samples taken for bile acid assay are collected only from a properly fasted animal. Even the sight or smell of food near the animal prior to blood collection can cause gall bladder constriction and invalidate the test results.

Dye clearance tests

The rate that the liver can excrete certain dyes provides a measure of the functional capabilities of the hepatocytes. The most commonly used dye in veterinary clinical medicine is bromsulphalein (BSP). For small animals, the dye is injected intravenously at a dosage of 5 mg/kg of body weight and becomes bound to albumin in the plasma. BSP dissociates from the albumin when it reaches the hepatocytes. In other areas of the body, capillaries are less permeable to proteins and the dye remains in the blood vessels. Most of the BSP which is taken up by hepatocytes is conjugated with glutathione and excreted into bile. Some BSP may remain unconjugated but is also excreted. After 30 minutes, a blood sample is taken and 1 ml of clear serum or plasma is placed in each of two tubes. The first tube is treated with 4 ml of 0.1N NaOH solution and inverted to mix. The second tube will serve as the instrument blank and is treated with 4 ml of 0.1N HCl. BSP color will be fully developed only in the alkaline solution. The blank tube is used to set the spectrophotometer to zero absorbance at 575 nm. The first tube is then read and its BSP concentration is obtained from a standard curve. The retention value is reported as the percentage remaining in the serum after 30 minutes. In healthy dogs, BSP retention of less than 5% is considered normal. In large animals, the procedure is similar, except that a pretest blood sample is taken and blood sampling requires serial determinations. Usually, two samples are taken at 4-minute intervals beginning 5 minutes after injection. Each sample is treated with the same reagent as that for small animals, except that 2 ml of serum is usually used for each 3 ml of reagent added. The pretest sample is used as the instrument blank. The BSP concentrations are determined from a standard curve and the results plotted against elapsed time on semi-logarithmic graph paper. Results are reported as the time required for serum BSP concentration to be halved. An example of a BSP clearance graph for large animals can be found in Fig. 6-3.

Enzyme analyses

Enzymes are specialized and very specific proteins which catalyze various chemical reactions. Most of the body's enzymes function intracellularly and are present in very low concentrations in serum. The reactants, referred to as substrates, bind to the enzyme, and this results in the formation of a product. The enzyme itself is not altered by or consumed during the reaction. Each specific enzyme usually catalyzes only one type of reaction. If an unlimited amount of substrate is available, the rate at which that substrate is consumed or product produced is a function of the amount of enzyme present. Measuring the consequences of enzyme activity then provides an indirect measurement of enzyme concentration. Enzyme assays represent a change per unit of time in a test system. The preferred unit of measure is the International Unit, abbreviated IU or U. The international unit is defined as the quantity of enzyme which will catalyze the reaction of one micromole of substrate to one micromole of product per minute under specific conditions. The test must be performed at the appropriate temperature and pH for that particular enzyme. A variety of test methodologies exists for serum enzyme analyses. Frequently, these assays report units different from the IU. The manufacturer of the reagent kit usually supplies the necessary conversion factor.

Enzyme assays may employ either an endpoint procedure or a kinetic procedure. The kinetic procedure involves monitoring the enzyme activity over a short period of time. Kinetic assays usually require a spectrophotometer capable of reading in the ultraviolet range. Endpoint procedures usually involve the addition of reagent to stop the reaction after a short period of time and then measuring the amount of enzyme activity.

Enzyme assays for liver function

Tests based on enzyme activity of hepatocytes are generally used as markers to detect liver damage rather than to distinguish specific functional defects. Depending on the species,

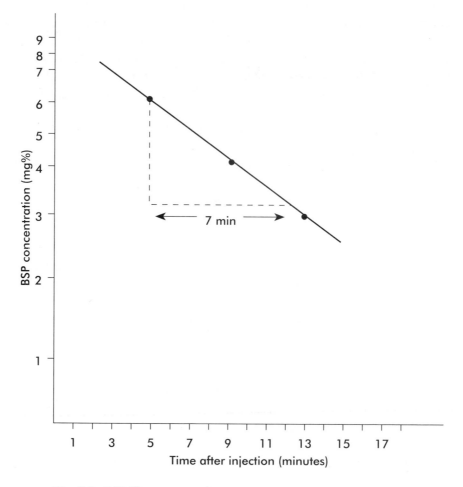

Fig. 6-3. BSP Clearance—equine.

enzymes frequently have multiple organ sources; that is, they are not always liver specific. Elevated levels of liver-specific serum enzymes are significant since these enzymes are produced and function within the hepatocytes. The enzyme may be attached to structures within the liver cell (e.g., mitochondria) or free in the cytoplasm. Damage to or necrosis of hepatocytes will result in the release of specific cellular enzymes into circulation. Other enzymes will be elevated primarily in response to obstructive disease.

Cellular enzymes of hepatocytes can be divided into four general groups: (1) phosphatases, (2) transaminases, (3) dehydrogenases, and (4) hydrolases. Most of these enzymes exist in several forms. These various forms are referred to as isoenzymes. A group of isoenzymes may demonstrate variability in specific functional parameters, such as temperature and pH. Hydrolase assays have limited application in veterinary medicine and are not routinely performed.

Phosphatases

This group of isoenzymes functions to catabolize organic phosphates. Blood contains two major groups of phosphatases, the alkaline phosphatases and the acid phosphatases. Care should be taken when collecting blood for phosphatase assay. The use of fluoride anticoagulants can inhibit phosphatase activity.

The acid phosphatases function at an optimum pH of 5. Acid phosphatase is released from lysed red cells and is found in bone and in the prostate. Determinations of acid phosphatase levels have limited value in veterinary medicine but can be useful in diagnosis of certain types of hemolytic anemia.

The alkaline phosphatases (AP) comprise a group of two isoenzymes, one of which has two isoforms. Alkaline phosphatases have multiple organ sources, including liver, kidney, and intestine, and function at an optimum pH of 9 to 10. Liver-specific alkaline phosphatase (LAP) and bone-specific alkaline phosphatase (BAP) are isoforms derived from a single gene. The two types differ in the extent of glycosylation. Intestinal alkaline phosphatase is another isoenzyme which is present in blood in very low levels. An additional type referred to as corticosteroid-induced alkaline phosphatase (CAP) is actually the intestinal form which may be converted to CAP following even small dosages of steroids.

With few exceptions, all isoenzymes of AP are present in very small amounts. Although it is possible to separate and quantify each individual fraction of AP with precipitation techniques, these procedures are rarely performed in veterinary practice. Significant increases in serum AP are almost always related to improper liver function. In the canine, increases of circulating levels of AP may indicate hepatic disease. The extent of such increase helps in differentiation of extrahepatic from intrahepatic insufficiency. Levels of AP 2 to 3 times normal are common in intrahepatic insult. Levels 10 to 15 times normal often indicate obstructive disease. These increases would be accompanied by increases in ALT levels (see next section). High levels (12 times normal) of serum alkaline phosphatases which are not accompanied by other abnormal liver function tests are often secondary to steroid administration.

The most commonly performed assay for serum alkaline phosphatase involves the use of a buffered phosphate-containing reagent which serves as a substrate for the AP. Phosphate ions are liberated in the reaction and reagent added to stop the reaction and to color the end product blue.

Transferases

Transferases are a group of enzymes that function to transfer amine groups from amino acids to keto acids, producing new amino acids. They are found primarily in tissues that have high rates of protein metabolism, especially kidney, liver, and muscle. In veterinary practice, the transaminases of clinical importance are alanine amino transferase (AL^T) and aspartate amino transferase (AST). Older literature may refer to these two enzymes as glutamic pyruvate transaminase (GPT) and glutamic oxalacetic transaminase (GOT), respectively. In dogs, cats, and primates, ALT is found in large amounts within the hepatocytes. Damage to hepatocytes results in release of large amounts of this enzyme. In other species, serum ALT levels are of little diagnostic value. AST is found in approximately equal amounts in both liver and muscle cells. AST assays are used primarily to estimate the extent of skeletal muscle damage in the equine and may be utilized to evaluate cardiac muscle damage in some species. Both AST and ALT assays involve the use of reagents which provide substrate for the enzyme. A colored end product is formed which is quantified in the spectrophotometer.

Ornithine carbamyl transferase and gamma glutamyl transferase are also liver-specific enzymes. Although evaluation of these enzymes may have some value in veterinary medicine, assay procedures are complicated and these tests are rarely performed.

Dehydrogenases

Dehydrogenases are a group of isoenzymes responsible for transferring hydrogen groups. They are cytoplasmic enzymes whose primary role is in glycolysis.

Lactic dehydrogenase (LDH)

Five different LDHs are present in a variety of tissues, including liver tissue. Any type of cell damage which results in a membrane defect will result in the release of LDH into surrounding tissue.

The most commonly performed assay for LDH is a kinetic procedure which indirectly measures LDH concentration by measuring the consumption of NAD. NAD functions in glycolysis as a cofactor for LDH. This assay is not considered liver specific unless the LDH fractions are first separated by electrophoresis. LDH assays have limited applications in veterinary medicine.

Sorbitol dehydrogenase (SDH)

Although present in a variety of organs, the greatest concentrations of SDH are found in the liver in most species. Lesser concentrations are found in kidney, small intestine, skeletal muscle, and erythrocytes. SDH functions as a catalyst for the conversion of polyhydric alcohol to glucose. SDH is the preferred assay to evaluate equine liver function. In the equine, serum SDH will show an immediate and marked increase in response to liver necrosis and usually returns to normal levels in less than 24 hours. SDH assays should be performed immediately after sample collection. The enzyme deteriorates rapidly at both refrigerator and room temperatures.

Glutamic dehydrogenase (GDH)

GDH is found bound to the mitochondria within the hepatocytes. Elevated serum levels of GDH are usually seen in only very severe liver disease. Although commercial test kits are not currently available, this is the enzyme of choice for evaluating bovine liver function.

Arginase

Arginase is found within the mitochondria of hepatocytes. Increases in serum arginase activity are diagnostic of liver necrosis in horses, cattle, pigs, and sheep. Elevations indicate severe liver damage. As liver tissue is regenerated, arginase levels quickly return to normal.

Kidney function tests

The kidneys have an important role in the homeostatic mechanisms of the body. They function to maintain the volume and composition of the extracellular fluid by selectively reabsorbing water and other essential constituents from the urinary filtrate. They are also involved in excretion of metabolic waste products and certain chemicals as well as functioning as an endocrine organ. The functional unit of the kidney is the nephron, which consists of a network of capillaries called the glomerulus and tubules which are lined with epithelial cells. The glomerular capillaries exhibit increased permeability as compared with capillaries found elsewhere in the body. Except for blood cells, large proteins, and fats, nearly all blood constituents pass through the glomerular membrane and enter the tubules. In a normally functioning nephron, about 80% of the water which passes through the glomerulus is reabsorbed in the tubules. Usually, all of the amino acids and glucose are also transported back across the tubular epithelium. Ions, such as sodium, chloride, and bicarbonate, are selectively reabsorbed by active transport. Since ions are charged molecules, reabsorption occurs either by exchanging an ion for a similarly charged molecule or by reabsorption of a pair of oppositely charged ions. Sodium may be exchanged for hydrogen, ammonium, or potassium ions. The selective reabsorption of ions is regulated by hormones. When properly functioning, these ion exchange systems help to maintain the constant pH of blood and body tissues. Those constituents which are not reabsorbed within the tubules are then excreted as urine. In addition, waste products may be secreted from tubule cells and enter the urine. Additional aspects of kidney function in urine formation will be discussed in Chapter 7.

Kidney damage may result in an inability of the glomerulus to retain cells and proteins or impaired reabsorption in the tubules. The nature and extent of this damage can be detected by either chemical analysis of the blood plasma or analysis of urine. In addition to the plasma proteins, a number of nonprotein nitrogenous (NPN) compounds are found in blood. These compounds include urea, creatinine, uric acid, and ammonia. NPN compounds are filtered through the glomerulus and some are partially reabsorbed in the tubules.

Urea nitrogen

The principal end product of protein catabolism is urea nitrogen. About half of the total NPN component of blood is urea nitrogen. Normally, all urea passes through the glomerular capillaries and enters the tubules. Normal passive diffusion processes result in the reabsorption of about 40% to 50% of the urea, with the remainder excreted in the urine.

Azotemia is an increase in urea nitrogen levels. Such increase can be due to multiple factors. Decreases in blood flow to the kidneys which alter the rate of filtration as well as obstructive disease within the urinary tract can affect urea nitrogen levels. A variety of infectious agents can also impair renal function by lysis of cells or accumulations of antigen-antibody complexes on the glomerular membrane.

Because of its low solubility, urea must be excreted in a relatively large volume of water. Dehydration will result in increased retention of urea in the blood. Excess protein intake as well as regular intense exercise results in increased production of urea. Differences in rates of protein catabolism between male and female animals, as well as young and adult animals, will also affect blood urea nitrogen levels.

A large variety of chemical reagent kits are available for urea nitrogen evaluations. These are primarily photometric procedures and the specific reagents used will vary depending on the manufacturer of the test kit. The Azostick is a dipstick procedure which can be used as a quick in-house screening test. The dipstick reacts with urea in blood, causing a color change on the stick. The intensity of that color is then visually matched with color standards. This method is less accurate than chemical assays. The potential for great error exists if standards are deteriorated or the technician's color vision is impaired.

Blood urea nitrogen measurements should be done in conjunction with creatinine measurements. Alteration in the ratio of urea nitrogen to creatinine is a more significant indicator of renal disease than are individual measurements of either component.

Creatinine

Creatinine is formed during normal muscle metabolism from the irreversible breakdown of creatine and creatine phosphate. The amount of creatinine present in serum is a function of the total muscle mass present. Creatinine is excreted by muscle cells at a relatively constant rate regardless of diet, age, or other factors. Normally, all plasma creatinine passes through the glomerular membrane and none is reabsorbed. A small amount of creatinine is also secreted by kidney tubule cells. Any condition which impairs glomerular filtration will result in increased serum creatinine levels.

The most commonly used method for measuring creatinine levels performed in veterinary clinical practice is the Jaffe spectrophotometric procedure. The Jaffe reaction utilizes a picric acid reagent at an alkaline pH. This reagent reacts with creatinine in serum, forming an orange-colored solution. A variety of test kits are available which contain slight variations in reagent content.

The creatinine clearance test is used as a measure of glomerular filtration. The test requires determinations of creatinine levels in both the urine and the serum, usually by utilizing the Jaffe reaction. The urine output in milliliters per minute, as averaged over several hours, is also needed. The creatinine clearance rate is then calculated with the following equation:

$$CCT = \frac{U \times V}{P} \times \frac{F}{A}$$

where U = mg/dl urine creatinine
P = mg/dl plasma creatinine
V = ml/min urine output

F/A represents a correction factor which is necessary to account for species variability. F is a species coefficient for the species being tested and A represents the body surface area in square meters.

Uric acid

Uric acid is a metabolic end product that is found mainly in the liver. The compound has low solubility and is usually transported to the kidney bound to albumin. Uric acid passes through the glomerulus but in most species is largely reabsorbed in the tubules. In primates and dalmation dogs, uric acid is not reabsorbed and is excreted in urine. In most mammals, however, the uric acid is reabsorbed and then oxidized to allantoin and other wastes. Photometric assays for uric acid are complicated and not routinely performed in veterinary clinical practice.

Pancreatic function tests

The majority of pancreatic tissue is associated with the production of digestive enzymes. This is referred to as the acinar function of the pancreas. The enzymes produced and their role in the digestive process are listed in Table 6-1. A small portion of pancreatic tissue is associated with the production of the hormones insulin and glucagon. Insulin affects all body cells by associating with specific cell receptors to allow the cell to take up glucose from the blood. Glucagon acts on hepatocytes and results in the conversion of stored glycogen to glucose.

Trauma to the pancreas is often assocaited with pancreatic duct inflammation. This results in a back-up of digestive enzymes into pancreatic capillaries and then into peripheral circulation. Evidence for damage to pancreatic tissue will frequently be seen as changes in fecal analysis. Undigested skeletal muscle fibers and fat may be evident in feces. A decrease in the body's concentration of fat-soluble vitamins may also be seen as the result of an impaired ability to digest lipids. In veterinary medicine, the most commonly used chemical tests of pancreatic function are serum assays for amylase, lipase, and glucose.

Serum amylase

Amylase functions as a catalyst in the breakdown of starch to glucose. A large variety of test methodologies is available in kit form. The specific test principle involved varies depending on the manufacturer of the kit. Like most enzyme analyses, amylase tests usually involve the addition of the substrate for the enzyme. Amylase activity may be measured by one of two general methods. Saccharogenic methods measure the total amount of alco-

TABLE 6-1

Major pancreatic enzymes

Enzyme	Digestive activity
Amylase	Carbohydrates
Lipase	Lipids
Nucleases	Nucleic acids
Chymotrypsinogen	Protein
Trypsinogen	Protein

hol-soluble sugar fragments that are released when serum amylase acts on a dyed starch substrate. Amyloclastic methods involve measurement of the disappearance of starch by utilizing a dye such as iodine to bind any unreacted starch in the system. The resulting colored complex can be quantified in the spectrophotometer.

Amylase is produced in tissues other than the pancreas, including salivary gland and small intestine. Amylase assay is therefore considered a less sensitive indicator of pancreatic function than lipase, which is derived solely from the pancreas.

Serum lipase

Nearly all serum lipase is derived from pancreatic acinar cells. Serum lipase analysis is therefore considered a specific indicator of pancreatic function. Lipase functions as a catalyst in the breakdown of triglycerides. Assays for serum lipase involve the addition of olive oil at a specific pH. In the presence of lipase, olive oil is hydrolyzed to glucose and fatty acids. The resulting suspension is measured spectrophotometrically.

Amylase and lipase assays provide the most valuable diagnostic information when serial determinations are made. Excess lipase is easily filtered through the kidney so lipase levels will remain normal early in pancreatic disease. Gradual increases in lipase levels are seen as disease progresses. With chronic, progressive pancreatic disease, the damaged pancreatic cells are replaced with connective tissue which cannot produce enzyme. A gradual decrease in both amylase and lipase levels will be seen.

Glucose

A small percentage of pancreatic cells are responsible for the production of the hormones glucagon and insulin. In the normal individual, insulin and glucagon levels are in relative equilibrium and blood glucose levels remain fairly constant. An increase in blood glucose is termed hyperglycemia. This condition can be caused by the presence of excess glucagon or by certain autoimmune diseases which result in the formation of anti-insulin antibodies. Excess of insulinase, an enzyme produced by the kidney to catabolize insulin, will also result in hyperglycemia. The highest blood glucose levels are seen in diabetes mellitus.

This disease is caused by a deficiency of insulin due to impaired pancreatic function that results in decreased or defective production of insulin.

Either decreased blood levels of insulin or defective production of insulin will reduce the ability of body cells to take up glucose from the blood. These higher blood glucose levels cannot be effectively reabsorbed by the nephron from the glomerular filtrate. Glycosuria (glucose in the urine) alters the solute concentration of the filtrate and leads to increased loss of electrolytes and nitrogen into the urine. Acids such as ketones, amino acids, and fatty acids are no longer being cycled through the normal glucose metabolic pathways and blood levels of these constituents increase. As the disease progresses, the body becomes unable to maintain the normal acid/base balance and blood pH increases.

Glucose assays

Several test methodologies are available in kit form for measurement of blood glucose levels. The sample required is usually either plasma or serum. Fluoride anticoagulants provide the best preservation of glucose but can interfere with some assays. Regardless of the test chosen, the sample should be processed quickly. If cells are allowed to remain in contact with the blood plasma or serum for an extended period, glycolysis will continue and glucose test results will be invalidated. Enzymatic assays are generally the most sensitive because they react only with glucose and not other sugars that may be present. However, these tests are sensitive to alterations in the test system. To provide accurate results, the assay must be performed at a specific temperature and pH. One commonly used kinetic assay involves the addition of glucose oxidase to the serum sample. This reacts with glucose in the serum to form gluconic acid and hydrogen peroxide. At an acid pH, peroxidase reacts with the hydrogen peroxide and chromogen in the test system and yields a red-colored end product which can be measured in the spectrophotometer. A second type of enzymatic assay has been developed recently. Hexokinase reagent catalyzes the reaction of glucose to glucose-6-phosphate (G-6-P). The addition of NADP+ to the system converts the G-6-P to glucose-6-phosphate dehydrogenase (G-6-PD) and produces NADPH. The amount of glucose present is thus proportional to the amount of NADPH produced.

Several types of endpoint assays are available for blood glucose analyses. These include the Benedict's copper reduction test and the σ-toluidine assay. Both of these involve the addition of reagent and chromogen, which react with glucose in the serum and create a colored end product. The specific product produced varies, but all can be measured spectrophotometrically. Some of these endpoint tests require the use of a boiling water bath. In addition, a variety of substances, such as other sugars and certain drugs, can interfere with the reactions. A thorough knowledge of the chosen test methodology is essential to providing reliable data.

A large variety of dedicated glucose instruments are available for use in the practice laboratory. Many of these were originally designed for use in human medicine to allow diabetic patients to monitor their own glucose levels. These instruments usually require only one drop of whole blood, placed on a dipstick. The color on the dipstick is read electronically. Although inexpensive and simple to use, correct procedure must be followed to ensure accuracy. The instrument must also be calibrated periodically with special control material. Dipstick glucose tests which are read visually are also available, but this method is subject to great error and is not recommended.

Glucose tolerance test

The results of a single blood glucose assay may help to identify any potential alterations in normal glucose metabolism. When these single test results are inconclusive, a glucose tolerance test is performed. This test is also performed to evaluate a diabetic patient's response to treatment or when adjustment of the patient's insulin therapy is needed. The glucose tolerance test (GTT) involves adminstration of glucose, either orally or intravenously. Samples for determination of blood glucose levels are taken immediately before and at specific time intervals after glucose is administered, usually every 30 to 60 minutes for 3 to 4 hours. Oral administration of glucose may be done in the dog. Ruminants do not respond to oral admninistration, and intravenous administration must be used.

The animal must be fasted for 24 hours before the test begins. A pretest sample for blood glucose analysis is taken. For the intravenous GTT test, a 50% solution of glucose is administered at the rate of 0.5 g/kg of body weight. The oral test is conducted by feeding a meal which contains glucose, 4 g/kg of body weight. If administered orally, blood glucose levels rise dramatically as the glucose is absorbed into the body. Peak blood glucose levels are usually reached in about 30 to 60 minutes. In normal animals, blood glucose levels then gradually decline to the pretest level by about the second hour of the test. A diabetic animal will usually still have high blood glucose levels at the completion of the test. Response to intravenous glucose administration will proceed in a similar manner, except that the initial rise will occur much more rapidly since the glucose does not have to be absorbed from the digestive tract.

Serum calcium

Although not a specific indicator of pancreatic function, serum calcium levels may be altered as a result of the acidosis found in many diabetic patients. In the normal animal, calcium levels remain relatively constant. The amount of calcium ingested daily is approximately equal to the amount excreted daily in urine. Nearly 99% of total body calcium is deposited in the skeletal system. Nonskeletal calcium is found both intracellularly and in the extracellular fluid.

Intracellular calcium is often bound to proteins of the mitochondria, cell membrane, or nucleus. Calcium in extracellular fluid plays a role in contraction of muscle, blood coagulation, enzyme activation, and transmission of nerve impulses. Plasma calcium is present in three forms. About half of the plasma calcium exists in a form that is bound to plasma proteins. A second portion exists as a complex bound to citrate. The remainder of plasma calcium consists of the ionic or free Ca^{+2}, which is the physiologically active form.

Measurement of only the ionized portion of plasma calcium is difficult and not routinely performed, except in research facilities. Methods to measure total serum calcium are performed on serum samples. Plasma is not suitable for analysis since most salt-based anticoagulants act by binding calcium and thus interfere with accurate analysis. The most commonly performed total serum calcium assay is a photometric procedure which utilizes a complexed cresolphthalein reagent. At an alkaline pH, this complex reacts with calcium to form a purple chromogen with maximum absorbance at 580 nm.

In addition to the effect of blood pH, calcium levels can be affected by a wide variety of factors. High plasma protein, some cases of hyperparathyroidism, and equine renal disease are all associated with increases in total serum calcium. When high calcium is present in conjunction with pancreatic necrosis, calcium may deposit in pancreatic tissue and serum calcium levels will decrease. Decreased serum calcium is also associated with deficiencies of vitamin D and protein.

Electrolytes

Electrolytes are ionic substances which are present in the body fluids. They function primarily in the regulation of the acid-base and osmotic balance of the body. The major electrolytes in plasma are sodium (Na^+), potassium (K^+), chloride (Cl^-), and bicarbonate (HCO_3^-).

Found primarily in extracellular fluid, sodium functions in the maintenance of plasma volume. Potassium concentration is greatest within the cells where it functions to regulate intracellular water balance. Chloride is an extracellular ion that functions in the regulation of electrolyte balance. Bicarbonate is primarily involved in the blood buffer system which regulates blood pH.

Techniques to measure electrolytes include chemical methods and ion-specific methods. Chemical methods are not routinely used since they measure all forms of the electrolyte rather than just those that are physiologically active. Ion-specific methods measure only the active (ionic) forms but require special instrumentation.

A flame photometer is a type of ion-specific analyzer which measures the wavelength emitted when ions are aspirated into a flame of a specific temperature. The instrument is similar in principle to the spectrophotmeter, except that a flame is used as the light source. Lithium is utilized as an internal standard and for comparison with the light emitted by the ions in the patient sample. The flame photometer can measure the concentration of both sodium and potassium simultaneously.

The development of ion-selective electrodes for many ions has greatly simplified electrolyte analyses. Instruments such as the Nova analyzer (Fig. 6-4) can provide accurate results in a few minutes and are self-calibrating. The analyzer utilizes potentiometric methods for specific ion measurements. In general, potentiometric analysis involves measurement of the electrical gradient between two areas. The two areas are separated by a membrane that is selectively permeable to a specific ion. An electrode that is also specific for that ion measures the change in electrical potential (voltage) as the ion diffuses through the membrane. This measurement is then compared to a reference electrode by an internal microcomputer. The degree of electrical potential change between the two electrodes is proportional to the number of specific ions present in the sample. The instrument measures this in millivolts and calculates the results in milliequivalents/liter. Specific electrodes are available for sodium, potassium, and chloride analyses that utilize this technology.

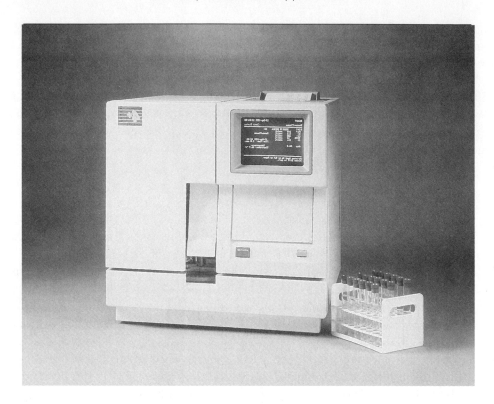

Fig. 6-4. Nova electrolyte analyzer. (Photo courtesy of Nova Biomedical.)

Alterations in acid-base balance are evaluated by measuring blood pH, P_{CO_2}, and bicarbonate levels. pH meters are readily available and easy to use. A number of automated instruments are available for blood gas, pH, and bicarbonate measurements. Most of these utilize potentiometric methods, although are few are photometric. Regardless of the instrument chosen, samples for pH and blood gas analysis must be carefully handled. Arterial blood samples are preferred. The sample must be collected in a manner which minimizes its exposure to air.

KEY POINTS

1. Instruments designed for clinical chemistry analysis employ either photometric or electrochemical principles.

2. Liver function tests are designed to measure serum concentrations of substances produced or processed by the liver or released by damaged hepatocytes.

3. Enzyme assays employ either endpoint or kinetic methodologies which measure enzyme activity, rather than concentration.

4. In veterinary medicine, liver-specific enzyme assays include tests for phosphatases, transaminases, and dehydrogenases.

5. Urea, creatinine, and uric acid are nonprotein nitrogenous compounds that are filtered through the kidney.

6. Glomerular filtration can be evaluated with the creatinine clearance test.

7. Renal disease may manifest as alteration in the ratio of blood urea nitrogen to creatinine in serum.

8. Acinar cells of the pancreas produce digestive enzymes, such as amylase and lipase.

9. A small portion of pancreatic tissue is responsible for the production of the hormones insulin and glucagon.

10. Since nearly all serum lipase is derived from the pancreas, lipase assay provides a more specific indicator of pancreatic function than amylase assay.

11. Insulin associates with specific cell receptors to increase the cell's permeability to glucose.

12. Enzyme assays for glucose are more sensitive than copper reduction or σ-toluidine assays.

13. Serum calcium levels can be affected by plasma protein concentration, blood pH, and deficiency of vitamin D.

14. Electrolytes are ions which function in regulating acid-base and water balance.

15. The major electrolytes in plasma are sodium, potassium, chloride, and bicarbonate.

16. Ion-specific electrodes are employed in potentiometric analyses of electrolytes.

REVIEW QUESTIONS

1. The Biuret procedure is used to measure _____ in serum.
2. Dye-binding methods are designed to measure the amount of _____ in serum.
3. Describe the metabolism of bilirubin in the normal animal.
4. Define "international unit."
5. List the enzyme assays used to evaluate liver function.
6. List the nonprotein nitrogen tests used to evaluate kidney function.
7. Define "azotemia."
8. List three factors that can affect blood urea nitrogen levels.
9. Creatinine is formed during _____ metabolism.
10. Uric acid is excreted in urine by primates and _____.
11. The production of digestive enzymes is referred to as the _____ function of the pancreas.
12. A small portion of pancreatic tissue is involved in the production of the hormones _____ and _____.
13. What effect does insulin have on body cells?
14. From what organs or tissues is amylase derived?
15. Which digestive enzyme is a more significant indicator of pancreatic function and why?
16. What is the principle behind the hexokinase assay for blood glucose?
17. In what forms can calcium exist in the blood?
18. The major electrolyte of intracellular fluid is _____.
19. Describe the principle of potentiometric analysis.

ANSWERS TO REVIEW QUESTIONS

1. The Biuret procedure is used to measure total protein in serum.
2. Dye-binding methods are designed to measure the amount of albumin in serum.
3. Bilirubin is carried to the liver loosely bound to albumin. Hepatocytes conjugate the bilirubin to glucuronic acid, forming bilirubin blucuronide, and this is secreted into bile. This is reduced to urobilinogen in the intestinal tract and then oxidized to urobilin.
4. An "international unit" is the quantity of enzyme required to catalyze the reaction of 1μ of substrate to 1μ of product in one minute, under specific conditions.
5. The enzyme assays used to evaluate liver function include AP, ALT, AST, and SDH.
6. The primary nonprotein nitrogen tests used to evaluate kidney function are blood urea nitrogen and creatinine. Uric acid may also be used in some species.
7. Azotemia refers to an increase in blood urea nitrogen levels.
8. The factors that affect blood urea nitrogen levels include blood pressure, obstruction within the urinary tract, and infectious diseases.
9. Creatinine is formed during muscle metabolism.
10. Uric acid is excreted in urine by primates and Dalmatian dogs.
11. The production of digestive enzymes is referred to as the acinar function of the pancreas.
12. A small portion of pancreatic tissue is involved in the production of the hormones insulin and glucagon.
13. Interaction with insulin increases a cell's permeability to glucose.
14. Amylase is derived from the pancreas, salivary gland, and small intestine.
15. Since all serum lipase is derived from the pancreas, lipase is a more specific indicator of pancreatic function than other digestive enzymes.
16. Serum glucose reacts with hexokinase to form G-6-P. This compound then reacts with NADP+ to produce G-6-PD and NADPH.
17. Calcium can exist in the blood in three forms: (1) Ca+ bound to plasma proteins, (2) Ca+ bound to citrate, and (3) ionic Ca^{+2}.
18. The major electrolyte of intracellular fluid is potassium.

19. Potentiometric analysis involves measurement of the electrical gradient between two areas which are separated by a membrane that is selectively permeable to a specific ion. An electrode that is also specific for that ion measures the change in electrical potential (voltage) as the ion diffuses through the membrane. This measurement is then compared to a reference electrode by an internal microcomputer. The degree of electrical potential charge between the two electrodes is proportional to the number of specific ions present in the sample.

SELECTED READING

Coles EH: *Veterinary Clinical Pathology*, ed 4. Philadelphia, 1986, WB Saunders Co.

Benjamin M: *Outline of Veterinary Clinical Pathology*, ed 3. Ames, IA, 1978, Iowa State University Press.

Carreiro-Lewandowski E, Duben-VonLaufen JL, Bishop ML: *Laboratory Manual for Clinical Chemistry*. Philadelphia, 1987, JB Lippincott.

Kaplan A, Szabo L: *Clinical Chemistry: interpretation and techniques*, ed 2. St. Louis, 1983, CV Mosby Co.

Tietz NW, editor: *Textbook of Clinical Chemistry*. Philadelphia, 1986, WB Saunders Co.

Kaplan LA, Pesce AJ: *Clinical Chemistry: theory, analysis, and correlation*. St. Louis, 1984, CV Mosby Co.

Mukherjee KL: *Review of Clinical Laboratory Methods*. St. Louis, 1979, CV Mosby Co.

Bishop ML, Duben-Engelkerk JL, Fody EP: *Clinical Chemistry: principles, procedures & correlations*. Philadelphia, 1992, JB Lippincott.

Calbreath DF: *Clinical Chemistry: a fundamental textbook*. Philadelphia, 1992, WB Saunders Co.

Wolf PL: *Practical clinical enzymology: techniques & interpretation*. 1982, RE Krieger Pub.

Urinalysis

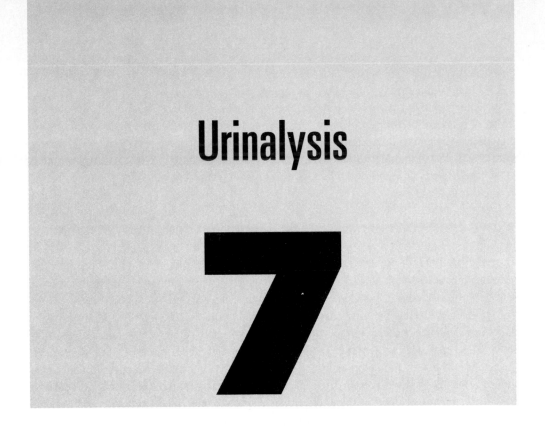

7

PERFORMANCE OBJECTIVES
After completion of this chapter, the student will:

Describe the functions of the various parts of the nephron in the formation of urine.

Explain the various methods of urine sample collection.

Describe the procedure for determination of specific gravity of a urine sample.

List the factors which can affect the color and clarity of a urine sample.

Describe the tests for urine glucose and
list the factors that may interfere with the test results.

List the advantages and disadvantages of urine dipstick tests.

Describe the procedures for chemical analysis of urine calcium and chloride.

Explain the procedure for preparation of a urine sample for microscopic analysis.

List the formed elements that may be found
in urine and their origin and possible significance.

Define the terms: hematuria, pyuria, hemoglobinuria, glucosuria, and proteinuria.

lthough numerous serum chemical assays are used as diagnostic tools by the clinician, urinalysis can provide perhaps the largest amount of diagnostic information. A properly performed urinalysis can provide data which aids in the evaluation of metabolic status, nutritional status, and kidney function. The kidneys are part of the urinary system which also includes the ureters, urinary bladder, urethra, and external urinary meatus. Urine is a physiologic fluid which is actively synthesized in the kidney from materials derived from the blood.

Formation of urine

The functional unit of the kidney is the nephron. Urine is formed by the filtration, selective reabsorption, and secretion of specific substances in specific locations within each nephron. The nephron consists of the glomerulus, Bowman's capsule, proximal convoluted tubule, Loop of Henle, distal convoluted tubule, and collecting tubule. The kidney also serves as an endocrine organ. Glandular tissue within the juxtaglomerular apparatus secretes the hormone angiotensinogen to help regulate blood pressure and thus the rate of filtration through the nephron. Each of the components of the nephron has a specific function in the formation of urine. The proper functioning of each component is vital in maintaining homeostasis in the organism. Regulation of water and electrolyte balance, blood pressure and pH, and elimination of waste are all affected by the kidney.

Filtration occurs between the glomerular capillary bed and Bowman's capsule. This process is accomplished by simple passive diffusion. The diffusion is driven by a pressure gradient between the capillaries and the permeable capsular membrane. The glomerulus has the highest pressure of any capillary bed. Under normal conditions, everything except blood cells and large molecular weight proteins (i.e., albumin and immunoglobulins) is filtered through the capsular membrane and enters the proximal convoluted tubule. Sodium, glucose, and other ions and nutrients are actively transported out of the filtrate in the proximal tubule and the Loop of Henle. Chloride ions and bicarbonate ions are reabsorbed by diffusion and some water is reabsorbed by osmosis. Within the distal tubule, additional sodium is removed from the filtrate and exchanged for hydrogen ions by active transport in response to the hormone aldosterone. Within both the distal tubule and the collecting tubule, ammonia, potassium ions, and hydrogen ions are secreted into the filtrate. Antidiuretic hormone released from the hypothalamus causes reabsorption by osmosis of vast amounts of water within the collecting tubule. The urine is then highly concentrated.

Specimen collection

Methods of sample collection must be chosen which will preserve the integrity of the sample and not interfere with test methodologies. Samples may be collected by catheterization, cystocentesis, or naturally. Natural collection provides a nonsterile sample and includes voluntary voiding of the bladder as well as manual compression. The sample should be collected midstream; that is, only after the first few milliliters have been voided. Care must be taken during collection so that contamination from organisms present around the external urinary meatus is avoided. Catheterization provides a sterile sample but is more difficult to obtain and poses a greater risk to the patient. Sterile equipment and technique must be used and catheter lubricants should be avoided as these will contaminate the sample. Cystocentesis can also provide a sterile sample and is the preferred method if urine bacterial cultures are needed. This poses the greatest risk for injury to the patient. Sterility of equipment and technique is crucial.

Types of samples

A first morning sample is generally the most desirable. This type of sample is usually the most concentrated and least affected by diet, water intake, and exercise. In some cases, formed elements will not be evident in the first morning sample and an additional sample from the patient's second void will be needed. Random samples, collected at various times throughout the day, are most convenient but show greatest variation in test parameters. In most cases, however, random samples are acceptable for microscopic analysis and most urine chemistry tests. When possible, a preprandial sample should be used. Postprandial samples show great variations due to dietary effects and may interfere with certain chemical assays which rely on color development. Samples collected over a 24 hour period can provide a true quantitation of the total kidney output per day.

Storage of samples

Samples should be immediately covered and taken to the laboratory for analysis (Fig. 7-1). If testing is to be delayed for more than one hour, precautions must be taken to maintain the integrity of the sample. Refrigeration will help to prevent bacterial overgrowth in the sample and reduce the possibility of destruction of formed elements in the urine. Chemical preservatives for urine are also available. These may be required if a sample is to be shipped for analysis. Many of these tablets, however, will interfere with certain urine chemistry assays. If samples are refrigerated, they must be warmed to room temperature and remixed before testing. The use of any chemical preservative must also be noted on the sample collection record.

PHYSICAL TESTING

As part of a routine urinalysis, the color, clarity, specific gravity, and pH of each urine sample should be evaluated.

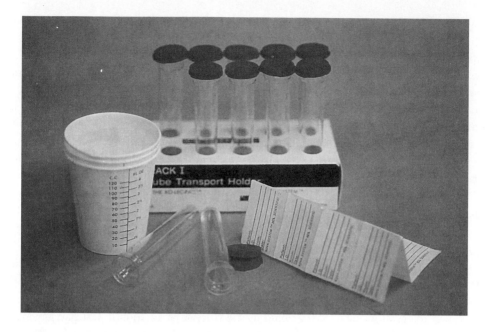

Fig. 7-1. Urine collection and processing containers.

Color

Although some species variability is evident, normal urine color is straw yellow. The intensity of the color depends upon the concentration of chemical constituents in the sample and the total volume of the sample. Higher volumes will result in more dilute urine, which is lighter in color. Administration of tetracyclines often results in an orange-colored urine. Certain foods, such as beets and asparagus, will also result in abnormal urine color. Red or brown urine may indicate the presence of blood or hemoglobin in the sample. Equine urine may turn brown if examination of the sample is delayed.

Clarity

In most species, urine is transparent. Cloudiness is considered normal in the rabbit and equine. Urine that has been refrigerated may become cloudy due to precipitation of dissolved materials. Gentle heating or the addition of a few drops of 5% acetic acid will clear the sample. If the urine does not clear, the degree of turbidity should be estimated, using a scale of slight to +4. Cloudy urine is primarily the result of an increase in the amount of microscopic material.

Specific gravity

Urine specific gravity (SG) is a measure of the amount of dissolved material present in the urine relative to distilled water. SG is a measure of the ability of the kidney to concentrate the urine. The primary solutes found in normal urine are sodium chloride and urea.

In small animal practice, SG values are usually obtained with a refractometer. The refractometer must be standardized with distilled water, which has an SG of 1.000. A few drops of well-mixed, room temperature urine are placed on the optical surface of the instrument and the hinged cover is then placed on top of the drops. The SG is read off the scale in the instrument.

A urinometer may also be used for SG determinations. The urinometer consists of a glass cylinder and a float, which must be periodically calibrated with distilled water. The glass apparatus should be filled about ¾ full with a well-mixed, room temperature sample. Avoid the formation of bubbles, especially on the top surface, as this will interfere with reading the results. The float is placed on top of the liquid, using a slight spinning motion. The urine SG is read off the scale of the urinometer at the bottom of the meniscus (Fig. 7-2).

Dilution of the urine sample may sometimes be required, especially if the volume of sample is not sufficient to fill the urinometer. Should dilution be required, the last two digits of the SG of the diluted sample are multiplied by the dilution ratio to yield the SG for the undiluted sample. For example, if 1 ml of urine sample is combined with distilled water to yield a total volume of 3 ml, the dilution ratio is 1:3. If the SG of this sample is now 1.010, then the SG of the undiluted sample is 1.030.

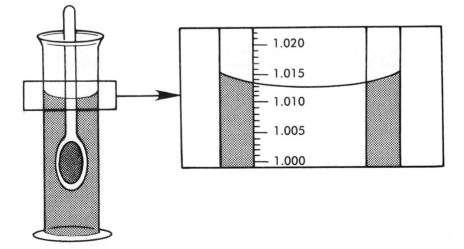

Fig. 7-2. The Urinometer is used for urine specific gravity measurements. The scale is read at the bottom of the meniscus.

Urine volume

The amount of urine produced per day is extremely variable. To properly quantify this volume, all urine voided over a 24 hour period is collected, beginning after the first morning sample on the first day of collection and ending with the inclusion of the first morning sample on the second day. Urine volume is affected by a large number of factors, including water intake, exercise, temperature, and body size.

An increase in daily urine output is termed polyuria. This is a common finding in patients that have diabetes mellitus, as well as a variety of renal diseases. Oliguria is a decrease in total urine volume and can be due to physiologic factors, such as decreased water intake. Oliguria can also be present in certain pathologic conditions, such as obstruction of renal flow.

Urine pH

pH is a measure of the hydrogen ion concentration of a solution. The ability of the kidneys to perform acid-base regulatory functions is reflected in urine pH. Carnivores and omnivores usually have acidic urine. Alkaline urine is characteristic of herbivores.

Methods to measure urine pH include pH hydrion paper and pH meters. Many urine dipstick tests incorporate pH portions with specific indicators for pH. These indicators are chemical substances which change color by reacting with hydrogen ions in urine. The color produced is visually compared to a color standard supplied with the dipstick.

Excess protein intake will increase urine acidity. The acidosis associated with diabetes mellitus will also result in increased acidity. Urine that is left at room temperature will gradually become more alkaline due to decomposition of urea in the sample.

CHEMICAL TESTING

The chemical constituents of urine that are of the greatest clincial importance include glucose, protein, bilirubin, urobilinogen, blood, and ketones. In the small veterinary practice, chemical testing is performed primarily by dipstick methods. A urine dipstick may be designed to test for a single chemical constituent or may have multiple test capabilities. The sticks contain pads that are impregnated with reagent (Fig. 7-3). Each pad contains a different reagent and addition of urine causes a color change on the pad. The color produced is compared with color standards supplied by the manufacturer.

Although these dipsticks are simple to use and provide results very quickly, the technician must ensure strict compliance with proper technique. As with all clinical testing, the sample must be collected and handled properly. A well-mixed, room temperature sample is required. The stick should be dipped briefly into the urine, ensuring that the reagent pad is fully immersed. Excess urine should be removed immediately. Each reagent pad is read at a specific time following immersion. Color development may continue on some test pads and

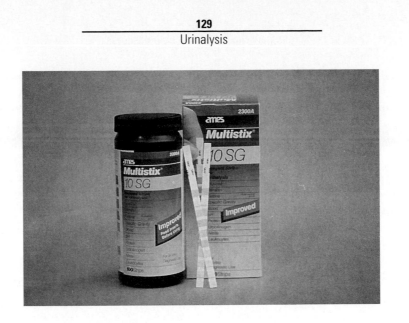

Fig. 7-3. A urine dipstick. The individual pads are impregnated with reagents which react with urine constituents.

results read after the recommended time may not be valid. It is crucial that the dipsticks be stored properly and the color standards not subjected to conditions which cause deterioration (e.g., sunlight, water). In some cases, dipstick tests provide only qualitative results; that is, they indicate only the presence or absence of a specific substance. Other tests may provide quantitative or semiquantitative results.

In additon to dipstick methods, a number of chemical tests exist which can detect and quantify protein, glucose, calcium, chloride, and other substances in urine.

Urine protein

Normally, all protein is reabsorbed in the kidney tubules and none is excreted. Globulins, which occasionally pass into urine, are not of clinical significance and do not usually react with most urine protein tests. The primary protein found in abnormal urine is albumin.

Protein measurements may be carried out by one of two methods. The sulfosalicylic acid test involves addition of reagent to the sample which causes precipitation of protein. The amount of protein in the sample is estimated by evaluating the degree of turbidity caused by the precipitation reaction. The reagent is available in tablet form (Bumintest tablets).

The Albustix protein test methodology is available either as a tablet or dipstick test. Both are colorimetric procedures which are similar, except for the type of buffer and indicator used. The buffer used for the tablet test is preferred for testing of alkaline urine samples. The procedure involves addition of one drop of urine to the tablet. This is allowed to absorb and then two drops of water are added. The color on top of the tablet following absorption of the water is compared to color standards supplied by the manufacturer.

Urine glucose

As with protein, all glucose is normally reabsorbed in kidney tubules. In certain disease conditions which are characterized by high blood glucose, glucose may not be completely reabsorbed and will be present in the urine (glucosuria).

Two types of urine glucose tests are commonly used: (1) the copper reduction test, and (2) the enzymatic test based on the glucose oxidase reaction. These tests are similar in principle to those described in the previous chapter for serum glucose. As with serum glucose, enzymatic tests tend to be more specific for glucose and less likely to react with other sugars that may be present in the urine.

Ketones

Ketones are intermediate compounds derived from the breakdown of fats. In the normal animal, minimal amounts of ketones are present in blood and urine. Any condition characterized by abnormal metabolism (e.g., diabetes mellitus) can result in increased levels of ketones in blood and urine. This condition is termed ketosis.

Most urine tests for ketones utilize the Ross methodology. This test involves a nitroprusside reagent which reacts with the ketones acetone and diacetic acid to form a purple-colored compound. The intensity of the color is compared with color standards supplied by the reagent manufacturer. Nitroprusside methods are used in both tablet and dipstick tests for ketones.

Blood

The presence of blood in the urine often indicates damage to the kidney or urinary tract. The ability to distinguish between the presence of red blood cells (hematuria) and the presence of free hemoglobin (hemoglobinuria) provides valuable diagnostic information. If the urine sample is not overly dilute or alkaline, centrifugation of the sample will force intact cells to sediment. Free hemoglobin will remain in the supernatant.

Bleeding in the urinary tract may occur in a variety of kidney disorders. Hematuria provides evidence for trauma to the urinary tract and is often seen in certain infectious diseases. Hemoglobinuria is a common finding in hemolytic diseases. It is important to distinguish true hemoglobinuria from in vitro hemolysis of red blood cells. Alkaline or dilute urines, in particular, may cause in vitro rupture of erythrocytes and subsequent release of hemoglobin.

Dipstick tests for blood include the Hemastix reagent strip. This dipstick incorporates a reagent which contains an organic peroxide. The presence of hemoglobin in the sample causes the reagent pad to change color. If intact cells are present, color will be present as spots on the reagent pad.

Bilirubin

Bilirubin is normally present in urine in small amounts that are undetectable with routine dipstick methods. Any disease which increases the amount of conjugated bilirubin in the blood will cause bilirubinuria. Unconjugated bilirubin is not water soluble and therefore not excreted in urine. Bilirubinuria is a common finding in the early stages of liver disease. Bilirubin usually appears in the urine before other signs of liver disease become apparent.

Dipstick and reagent tablet tests are available for determination of urine bilirubin. These utilize a reagent which contains a diazo component that reacts with bilirubin to produce a color change.

Urobilinogen

Urobilinogen is a normal end product of bilirubin metabolism and is present in small amounts in urine. Decreases in the amount of urine urobilinogen may indicate obstruction of the bile passages. Increased amounts of urine urobilinogen are associated with a variety of hepatic and hemolytic diseases.

Tests for urine urobilinogen utilize a benzaldehyde reagent which reacts with urobilinogen to form a colored compound.

Calcium

Alterations in urine calcium are seen frequently in chronic renal disease. The most commonly used assay for urine calcium is the Sulkowitch semiquantitative test. Sulkowitch reagent contains ammonium oxalate, which reacts with calcium to form an insoluble precipiate. The test is performed by diluting 5 ml of urine with 5ml of distilled water. In a second tube, equal amounts of urine and Sulkowitch reagent are combined. The two tubes are compared at 2 and 10 minutes for evidence of precipitation. Results are recorded as "low" if no visible precipitation is present. A normal result is demonstrated by a fine white cloud of precipitate. A heavy, white precipitate indicates high urine calcium.

Chloride

A decrease in urine chloride is an early indicator of salt depletion and is also seen in potassium deficiency. Urine chloride is measured with the Fantus method. The test is performed by placing ten drops of urine in a test tube and adding one drop of 20% potassium chromate solution. A 2.9% solution of silver nitrate is then added dropwise, agitating the tube after each drop is added. When all available urine chloride has reacted with the silver nitrate, the excess silver nitrate will react with the potassium chromate and form a red silver chromate precipitate. Chloride concentration is calculated by multiplying the number of drops of silver nitrate used by one thousand to give results in mg/liter. This can be converted to milliequivalents/liter by multiplying by 0.0171.

Bacteria

Many types of bacterial organisms can infect the urinary tract. The majority of these are gram negative organisms that contain enzymes to reduce nitrate to nitrite. Dipstick reagents for nitrate-reducing bacteria undergo color change when the levels of these bacteria are greater than 10^5 per milliliter. Samples for bacterial dipstick analysis must be collected aseptically and tested as soon as possible.

Leukocytes

The presence of abnormally high numbers of leukocytes in urine is termed pyuria. A significant increase in leukocyte numbers indicates urinary tract infection. Neutrophils, in particular, will enter the glomerular filtrate in an attempt to combat the infection. Neutrophilic granules contain enzymes that can be detected with chemical dipstick tests. Any positive result for leukocytes on a dipstick test should be confirmed with microscopic analysis of the sample.

Automated systems

Analyzers designed to perform automated urinalysis are of great value in the busy veterinary clinical laboratory (Fig. 7-4). These instruments are capable of performing complete urine profile on multiple samples in just a few minutes. The test methodologies employed are the same as those used for dipstick analysis. In many cases, the dipstick is a component of the analyzer and is read electronically rather than visually. Some of these instruments have computer software which provide printed results and maintain several hundred urinalysis profiles in memory.

MICROSCOPIC EXAMINATION

Microscopic examination of urine sediment may be necessary to assist the clinician in differential diagnosis or to follow the course of renal disease. The type of sediment present can help to distinguish renal from postrenal abnormalities. Normal urine contains little or no sediment.

Formed elements

The formed elements found in urine include cells, crystals, and casts (see the box on page 134). Casts are structures formed in renal tubules from protein precipitate of disintegrating tubule cells.

Accurate urine microscopic analysis requires strict adherence to proper technique. Errors in collection or processing of the sample will introduce variables which may render the data useless. A freshly voided sample is essential. Random samples must be avoided as the more dilute urine characteristic of a random sample may cause lysis of cellular ele-

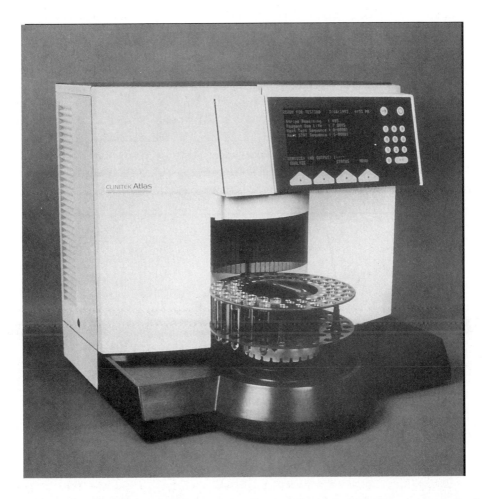

Fig. 7-4. A urine dipstick reader. This instrumentation provides a more accurate assessment of color changes on urine dipsticks than a visual assessment done by the technician. (Photo courtesy Miles Inc., Diagnostics Division.)

ments. A clean collection container must be used and the sample collected in a manner that minimizes contamination with cellular debris from the urethral meatus. The collection vessel must be immediately covered and microscopic examination done without delay. The procedure for preparation of the urine for sediment examination is as follows:

1. Fill a conical centrifuge tube with 10 ml of a well-mixed urine sample.
2. Cap the tube and centrifuge at 2000 RPM for 8 to 10 minutes, preferably at controlled refrigerator temperature.
3. Carefully pour off the supernatant, leaving about 1 ml of material in the bottom of the tube.
4. Gently resuspend the sediment in the remaining urine using a Pasteur pipette.
5. Set up two wet mounts by placing two drops of the resuspended urine, side by side, on a clean glass slide.
6. Add one drop of stain (Sedi-Stain) to one of the drops.
7. Add a large rectangular coverslip to cover both drops.

   The slide is then examined under the low-power lens for evidence of casts. Other elements will be found by using the high-power lens. Any formed elements found in the sample should be counted and the count averaged over ten microscopic fields. Both the stained and the unstained preparations should be examined. Staining can interfere with identification of certain elements but may help in cell identification. Use of a phase contrast microscope is preferred for evaluating unstained sediment.

Formed elements in urine sediment

I. Cells
  A. Blood cells
    (1) Erythrocytes
    (2) Leukocytes
  B. Epithelial cells
    (1) Squamous
    (2) Transitional
    (3) Renal tubule
II. Casts
  A. Hyaline
  B. Cellular
    (1) RBC casts
    (2) WBC casts
    (3) Epithelial casts
  C. Granular
  D. Waxy/fatty

III. Crystals
  A. Normal
    (1) Acid urine
      (a) Uric acid
      (b) Potassium urate
    (2) Acid to Neutral Urine
      (a) Hippuric acid
      (b) Calcium oxalate
    (3) Alkaline urine
      (a) Calcium carbonate
      (b) Triple phosphate
      (c) Ammonium urate
  B. Abnormal (Acid urine)
    (1) Sulfamerazine
    (2) Bilirubin
    (3) Cholesterol
    (4) Leucine
    (5) Tyrosine

Cells

The cellular elements found in urine sediment include epithelial cells, erythrocytes, and leukocytes. Bacteria and certain infectious agents may also be found.

Epithelial cells are of three types. Those derived from the urethra and the bottom third of the bladder wall are squamous epithelial cells. These are found in nearly all normal urine sediment and are not a significant indicator of pathology. Transitional epithelial cells are derived from the upper portion of the bladder, ureter, and pelvis of the kidney. They may be of variable shapes, from round to oval or caudate. The presence of transitional epithelial cells is significant if they are present in large numbers. Renal tubule cells are small round cells with a single nucleus and their presence usually indicates active degeneration of renal tubules.

Erythrocytes should not be present in normal urine, especially if measures to reduce contamination have been followed. The presence of more than three red blood cells per high-power field usually indicates an abnormal condition. Erythrocytes in concentrated urine may be crenated. Red blood cells usually will lyse in alkaline or dilute urine. If the sample was collected by catheterization, some red blood cells may be expected. The appearance of the red blood cell will vary. They are sometimes yellow or orange colored and may be colorless.

Leukocytes in urine are also called pus cells. They appear as granular cells and often have degenerating nuclei. A few leukocytes may be found in normal urine. If large numbers are found, infection of the urinary tract is likely.

Infectious agents, especially gram-negative bacteria, may sometimes be found. Bacteria may appear motile and staining may help to identify the particular type of organism. If the sample was collected aseptically, no bacteria should be present. Large numbers of bacteria may indicate urinary tract infection, especially if found in conjunction with pyuria. Other infectious agents, such as *Trichomonas*, *Balantidium*, *Entamoeba*, and ova of parasites are usually contaminants of the sample.

Crystals

The specific type of urine crystals found varies with the pH of the urine. Some of these crystals are formed as the urine cools. Amorphous crystalline materials are generally of no clinical significance. Crystals that may be found in normal acid urine include uric acid, amorphous urates, and potassium urate. In acid to neutral pH urine, hippuric acid and calcium oxalate are normally seen. In alkaline urines, calcium carbonate, triple phosphate, ammonium urate, and amorphous phosphates are common. The technician must become familiar with the appearance of these crystals. The physical characteristics of a particular urine crystal will vary and the technician must become familiar, with experience, in identifying these normal variations.

Abnormal crystals are not present in alkaline or dilute urine. Abnormal crystals found in acid urine include bilirubin, cholesterol, leucine, cystine, tyrosine, and sulfamerazine.

Leucine and tyrosine are seen in acute liver disease. Cystine crystals form as a result of impaired protein metabolism. In cases of urolithiasis, it is essential to properly identify urine crystals. Ideally this identification should be done by attempting to dissolve the crystal in different solutions. The type of solution which is capable of dissolving the crystal allows for identification.

Casts

Casts are formed as tubule cells disintegrate. These disintegrating cells release protein precipitate that takes on the shape of the renal tubule. Casts are large structures and are usually present in undetectable amounts. The presence of large numbers of casts indicates pathologic renal tubule degeneration. Casts are formed primarily in the distal and collecting tubules. Ideal conditions for cast formation are acid urine, slowly moving filtrate, and high salt and protein concentration. Casts are named according to the specific inclusions found in them.

Hyaline casts are composed only of protein. They are colorless, semitransparent, and usually have rounded ends. Granular casts are hyaline casts that contain granules derived from disintegrating tubular epithelium. These are further subdivided into coarse granular and fine granular casts. Fatty and Waxy casts are broader than hyaline casts and contain globules that appear refractile. Cylindroids are actually partially formed hyaline casts that have one tapered end. Blood casts appear as deep red- or orange-colored homogeneous hyaline casts. Cellular casts may contain red blood cells or pus cells. Each type of cast is associated with a particular defect in a specific portion of the renal tubule. Every attempt must be made to properly identify casts in urine samples to aid the clinician in correct diagnosis.

Other elements

A variety of other elements are found in urine. Mucus and mucin threads are common, especially in normal horse urine. Yeast and fungi may be seen and are usually present as contaminants.

KEY POINTS

1. Urine is a physiologic fluid that is actively synthesized by the kidney using materials derived from blood.

2. The functional unit of the kidney is the nephron which consists of the glomerulus, Bowman's capsule, proximal convoluted tubule, Loop of Henle, distal convoluted tubule, and collecting tubule.

3. Regulation of water and electrolyte balance, blood pressure and pH, and elimination of waste are all affected by the kidney.

4. Urine specimen collection methods include catheterization, cystocentesis, and natural voiding.

5. Random samples are less desirable than the more concentrated first morning sample.

6. First morning samples show the least variation due to diet, exercise, and other factors.

7. Physical testing of urine includes evaluation of urine color, clarity, specific gravity, pH, and volume.

8. Urine specific gravity is a reflection of the ability of the kidney to concentrate the urine and is usually tested with a refractometer or urinometer.

9. Urine volume is best evaluated with a 24 hour sample.

10. Urine pH is a measure of the hydrogen ion concentration of the urine and reflects the ability of the kidney to maintain acid-base balance.

11. Chemical testing of urine includes qualitative and/or quantative assays for glucose, protein, bilirubin, urobilinogen, blood, and ketones.

12. Most urine chemical testing is performed with dipstick methods.

13. Protein, glucose, and blood should not be present in urine samples from normal patients.

14. Hematuria is the presence of intact red blood cells in urine and must be distinguished from hemoglobinuria, which is the presence of free hemoglobin in the urine.

15. The Sulkowitch test provides a semiquantitative measure of urine calcium.

16. The Fantus method is used to measure the amount of chloride present in urine.

17. Microscopic examination of urine sediment can provide valuable diagnostic infor-mation. Careful attention to proper technique will help ensure accurate results.

18. The formed elements in urine sediment that may be found microscopically include bacteria, epithelial cells, blood cells, casts, and crystals.

REVIEW QUESTIONS

1. Define "urine."
2. What role does the juxtaglomerular apparatus play in the formation of urine?
3. In what part of the nephron is the greatest amount of water reabsorbed?
4. Why is a first morning urine sample preferred to a random sample?
5. What is the significance of brown-colored urine?
6. If a urine sample is diluted 1:2 and the specific gravity of the diluted sample is 1.005, what is the actual SG of the sample?
7. The tablet Albustix test for protein is preferred when the sample has an _____ pH.
8. Define "hematuria" and "hemoglobinuria."
9. The Ross methodology is used to test for _____ in urine.
10. The Sulkowitch test is used to estimate the concentration of _____ in a urine sample.
11. Describe the principle behind the Fantus test for urine chloride.
12. The presence of greater than _____ bacteria per ml of sample indicates the possibility of urinary tract infection.
13. Describe the procedure for preparation of urine sediment for microscopic analysis.
14. List the three types of epithelial cells that may be found in urine.
15. Abnormal crystals are not present in urine that has an _____ pH.
16. List the normal crystals found in acid urine.
17. List the normal crystals found in alkaline urine.
18. What are "casts" and how are they formed?

ANSWERS TO REVIEW QUESTIONS

1. Urine is a physiologic fluid that is actively synthesized by the kidney using materials derived from blood.
2. The juxtaglomerular apparatus secretes hormone which alters blood pressure and, therefore, the flomerular filtration rate.
3. The greatest amount of water is reabsorbed within in the collecting tubules.
4. A first morning urine sample is least affected by dietary factors and usually adequately concentrated so that formed elements remain intact.
5. Brown-colored urine may indicate the presence of blood. In the equine, brown urine may indicate that oxidation processes have occurred in the urine sample.
6. If a urine sample is diluted 1:2 and the specific gravity of the diluted sample is 1.005, the actual SG of the sample is 1.010.
7. The tablet Albustix test for protein is preferred when the sample has an alkaline pH.
8. Hematuria is the presence of intact red blood cells in urine. Hemoglobinuria is the presence of free hemoglobin.
9. The Ross methodology is used to test for ketones in urine.
10. The Sulkowitch test is used to estimate the concentration of calcium in a urine sample.
11. When all available urine chloride has reacted with the silver nitrate, excess silver nitrate will react with potassium chromate and form a red silver chromate precipitate. Chloride concentration is calculated by multiplying the number of drops of silver nitrate used by one thousand to give results in mg/liter.
12. The presence of greater than 10^5 bacteria per ml of sample indicates the possibility of urinary tract infection.
13. For preparation of urine sediment for microscopic analysis: (1) Fill a conical centrifuge tube with 10 ml of well mixed urine. (2) Cap the tube and centrifuge at 2000 RPM for 8 to 10 minutes. (3) Carefully pour off the supernatant, leaving about 1 ml of material in the bottom of the tube. (4) Gently resuspend the sediment in the remaining urine using a Pasteur pipette. (5) Set up two wet mounts by placing two drops of the resuspended urine, side by side, on a clean glass slide. (6) Add one drop of stain (Sedi-Stain) to one of the drops. (7) Add a large rectangular coverslip to cover both drops.
14. The three types of epithelial cells that may be found in urine include: (1) squamous epithelial cells derived from the urethra and the bottom third of the bladder wall, (2) transitional epithelial cells derived from the upper portion of the bladder, ureter, and pelvis of the kidney, and (3) renal tubule cells.

15. Abnormal crystals are not present in urine that has an alkaline pH.
16. Normal crystals found in acid urine include uric acid, potassium urate, hippuric acid, and calcium oxalate.
17. Normal crystals found in alkaline urine include calcium carbonate, triple phosphates, and ammonium urate.
18. Casts are formed elements found in urine that are derived from disintegrating renal tubule cells. Protein precipitate released by these cells takes the shape of the tubule.

SELECTED READING

Ames Division, Miles Diagnostics: *Modern Urine Chemistry*. Elkhart, Indiana, 1987, Mile Laboratories, Inc.

Osborne CA, Stevens JB: *Digest of Canine and Feline Urine Sediments*. St. Louis, 1979, Ralston Purina Co.

Strasinger SK: *Urinalysis in Clinical Laboratory Practice*. Cleveland, 1975, CRC Press.

Coles EH: *Veterinary Clinical Pathology*, ed 4. Philadelphia, 1986, WB Saunders.

Benjamin M: *Outline of Veterinary Clinical Pathology*, ed 3. Ames, IA, 1978, Iowa State University Press.

Mukherjee KL: *Review of Clinical Laboratory Methods*. St. Louis, 1979, CV Mosby Co.

Graff L: *A Handbook of Routine Urinalysis*. Philadelphia, 1983, JB Lippincott.

ROCOM Press: *Urine Under The Microscope*. Nutley, NJ, 1973, Hoffman-LaRoche Inc.

Haber MH: *Urinary Sediment: a textbook atlas*. Chicago, 1981, American Society of Clinical Pathology.

Glossary

absolute value   measure of the actual numbers of each leukocyte type in a microliter of blood. Calculated by multiplying the number of leukocytes by the relative percentage of each leukocyte type obtained from the differential count.

acanthocyte   an erythrocyte with spiny projections.

acidosis   pathologic decrease in pH due to accumulation of acids or decrease in bicarbonate concentration in blood and body tissues.

accuracy   the closeness with which a measured value approaches its true value.

agglutination   clumping of particles (e.g., blood cells) by antibody specific for the particles.

agranulocyte   a white blood cell without obvious cytoplasmic granules.

albumin   the principle protein of blood plasma which functions in the maintenance of osmotic balance in the body.

aldosterone   hormone secreted by the adrenal cortex which increases retention of sodium (and therefore water) and the excretion of potassium.

allergy   see Hypersensitivity.

amino transferases   enzymes that catalyze the transfer of amine groups.

amylase   enzyme that catalyzes the fragmentation of starch.

anemia   a decrease in oxygen-carrying capacity of blood.

angiotensin   compound which stimulates aldosterone secretion, raises blood pressure, and reduces kidney flow.

anisocytosis   abnormal variation in erythrocyte size.

antibody   specialized and specific protein produced by B-lymphocytes in response to an antigen.

anticoagulant   substance that inhibits or prevents blood clotting.

antigen   any substance which is capable of eliciting a response from the immune system.

anulocyte   bowl-shaped erythrocyte.

artifact   any variation in normal appearance of a structure or measurement of a substance that is caused by improper technique.

assay   measurement of the amount of a specific constituent in a mixture of substances.

autoimmunity   any condition that results in production of antibody against a body's own tissues.

B-cell   lymphocyte which is capable of secreting antibody.

band cell   immature leukocyte.

Barr body   small, dense chromatin mass found in cells from female organisms; represents inactive X chromosome.

basket cell   in hematology, a degenerative or ruptured cell.

basophilia   bluish appearance of cells or cell constituents as a result of affinity to basic dyes.

Beer's law   relationship between concentration of a substance and its absorbance and transmission of monochromatic light: absorbance is directly related to concentration in a linear fashion; transmission is inversely and logarithmically related to concentration.

bilirubin   orange-colored insoluble pigment produced by the breakdown of heme.

bilirubin glucuronide   soluble, conjugated form of bilirubin secreted by hepatocytes.

blast cell   any immature cell which represents a precursor in the development of a particular cell line.

buffy coat layer of material above the packed erythrocytes following centrifugation; consists of leukocytes, thrombocytes, and sometimes nucleated erythrocytes.

carboxyhemoglobin irreversible and useless form of hemoglobin which has bound to carbon monoxide.

cast structure formed by protein precipitate of degenerating kidney tubule cells which takes the shape of the tubule; may contain cellular elements.

coagulation factor one of several blood proteins which are required for normal activation of the blood clotting pathways.

complement series of plasma proteins that interact with cells and molecules of the immune system.

control biologic substance used in quality control programs to verify correct operation of test systems.

creatinine nonprotein nitrogenous substance produced as an end product of normal muscle metabolism and excreted through the kidneys.

crenation scalloped edge appearance of a cell which has been exposed to hypertonic conditions; artifact of erythrocytes produced by slow drying of a blood smear.

cyanmethemoglobin hemoglobin produced as a result of exposure to certain forms of cyanide; used in the assay procedure for blood hemoglobin determination.

dehydrogenases group of enzymes that catalyze the transfer of hydrogen groups.

differential hematologic test for determining the relative percentages of each leukocyte type as present on a blood smear.

Döhle body small gray-blue patches of cytoplasm seen in some immature granulocytes; represent ribosomes.

donut cell artifact produced by excess pressure on a cell which causes the center of the cell to punch out.

electrolyte any substance which dissociates into ions when dissolved in water. In clinical medicine, those ions which play a role in acid-base and water balance—sodium, potassium, chloride, and bicarbonate.

ELISA enzyme-linked immunosorbent assay; an immunologic test designed to demonstrate the presence or absence of a specific antigen or antibody.

enzyme specialized and specific proteins which act as catalysts in various chemical reactions and are regenerated in an unchanged form.

erythrocyte indices calculated values which provide the average volume and hemoglobin concentration of the erythrocytes in a blood sample.

erythropoiesis the production of erythrocytes.

erythropoietin hormone secreted by the kidney which acts to stimulate erythropoiesis in bone marrow stem cells.

ESR erythrocyte sedimentation rate; a measure of the speed with which erythrocytes fall in their own plasma under specific conditions.

fibrin insoluble plasma protein formed from the action of thrombin on fibrinogen; essential for blood clotting.

fibrinolysis enzymatic dissolution of a fibrin clot.

fixative substance capable of maintaining normal appearance and chemical composition of cells and tissues; used to preserve specimens.

flame photometer instrument designed for analysis of chemical substances which measures the wavelength of light emitted by the substance under specific conditions.

gamma globulins group of plasma proteins that function primarily in the immune response; immunoglobulins.

glucose monosaccharide that represents the end product of carbohydrate metabolism; storage form of energy.

glucose-6-phosphate dehydrogenase   enzyme catalyst found in erythrocytes; allows for the oxidation and reduction of hemoglobin as the hydrogen carrier in glycolysis.

hapten   small molecule that is antigenic only when attached to a larger carrier protein.

Heinz body   erythrocyte inclusion that represents denatured hemoglobin.

hemoglobinuria   presence of hemoglobin in the urine.

hematopoiesis   production of blood cells.

hematuria   presence of intact red blood cells in the urine.

hemoglobin   erythrocyte protein which acts as a carrier molecule to bring oxygen to tissues and carbon dioxide to lungs.

hemolysis   destruction or fragmentation of erythrocytes.

hemostasis   maintenance of the integrity of the blood and blood vessels.

homeostasis   maintenance of the state of constancy of the body's internal environment.

hyperchromic   abnormal increase in the intensity of a cell's characteristic staining pattern.

hypersensitivity   an abnormal increased immune system response.

hypertonic   a substance or fluid having a solute concentration less than that in which it is contained.

hypochromic   abnormal decrease in the intensity of a cell's characteristic staining pattern.

hypotonic   a substance or fluid having a solute concentration greater than that in which it is contained.

icterus   see jaundice.

ion   any molecule which has a positive or negative charge as a result of gaining or losing electrons.

isotonic   a condition in which two substances or fluids have equal solute concentration so that the net movement of water between them is equal.

jaundice   abnormal yellowish discoloration of skin, mucous membrane, or blood plasma as a result of an increase in bile pigments.

karyorrhexis   rupture of the nucleus of a cell.

karyolysis   degeneration or dissolution of the nucleus of a cell.

kinetic assay   a chemical test which measures the rate of change of a substance in the test system.

leptocyte   an erythrocyte with a decrease in volume relative to its diameter.

leukocytosis   an increase in the number of circulating white blood cells.

leukopenia   a decrease in the number of circulating white blood cells.

leukopoiesis   the production of white blood cells.

lipase   enzyme which catalyzes the breakdown of fats.

lipemia   presence of excess fatty material in blood plasma or serum.

lysis   destruction.

macrocyte   erythrocyte with an abnormally large diameter.

macrophage   phagocytic cell derived from the blood monocyte.

megakaryocyte   large bone marrow cell which gives rise to blood platelets.

microcyte   erythrocyte with an abnormally small diameter.

morphology   appearance of a cell or tissue.

NK cell   natural killer cell; cell that is capable of direct attack on an antigen without specificity for the antigen.

neutralization   antigen-antibody interaction that renders an antigen nonfunctional.

neutropenia   a decrease in the absolute number of circulating neutrophils.

neutrophilia   an increase in the absolute number of circulating neutrophils.

opsonization   an antigen-antibody interaction which increases an antigen's susceptibility to phagocytosis.

osmotic fragility   measure of the susceptibility of the erythrocyte to lysis in solutions of varying osmotic concentration.

ovalocyte   an oval or elliptical erythrocyte.

oxyhemoglobin   hemoglobin that is bound to oxygen.

pH   measure of the hydrogen ion concentration of a solution.

phagocyte   any cell that is capable of ingesting particles or organisms.

phosphatases   group of enzymes that catalyze the reaction of organic phosphates.

plasma   the liquid portion of the blood.

plasma cell   a B-lymphocyte that has differentiated to an antibody-secreting cell.

poikilocyte   an abnormally shaped cell.

polychromasia   variation in the staining pattern of a cell.

polycythemia   an increase in the number of circulating erythrocytes.

polyuria   an increase in the volume of urine voided per day.

potentiometer   an instrument which utilizes an ion-selective electrode to measure the difference in electric potential as a function of the amount of the specific ion present in a sample.

precipitation   a reaction which results in the formation of insoluble particles which settle out of a solution.

precision   measure of the reproducibility of a test.

pyuria   presence of abnormally large numbers of leukocytes in urine.

quality control   laboratory program designed to ensure the accuracy and precision and thus reliablility of test results.

refractive index   measure of the degree of light bending as it passes from one media to another, relative to air.

reticulocyte   an anuclear, immature erythrocyte.

rouleaux   arrangement of red blood cells in a column that resembles a stack of coins.

schistocyte   an erythrocyte that has fragmented.

serum   the liquid portion of blood which remains after the blood has been allowed to clot; contains all plasma constituents except those involved in coagulation.

smudge cell   a leukocyte that has ruptured; basket cell.

specificity   measure of the ability of a molecule to react with only a specific molecule.

spectrophotometer   instrument designed to measure the amount of monochromatic light which is absorbed or transmitted when passed through a substance.

spherocyte   a small round erythrocyte with a decrease in diameter relative to cell volume.

stab cell   see band cell.

stomatocyte   an erythrocyte with a linear area of pallor.

T-cell   a group of related lymphocytes which mature in the thymus and function in the immune system.

target cell   a leptocyte with a peripheral ring of cytoplasm surrounded by a clear area and a dense central rounded area of pigment.

titer   dilution at which a sample no longer yields a positive result for specific antigen or antibody.

toxic neutrophil   a neutrophil with abnormal granulation, basophilic cytoplasm, vacuoles, or condensed nuclear chromatin.

urea nitrogen   an end product of protein metabolism formed in the liver.

uric acid   an end product of nucleic acid metabolism in some species.

veterinary technician   a dedicated, tireless and vital member of the veterinary medical team; person with a minimum of 2 years of specialized college training who performs myriad technical procedures in the veterinary hospital; saint.

The data on the following pages was compiled from a variety of sources including workshops, personal notes, and the references listed at the end of each chapter. Normal values can be affected by a large number of factors such as the type of equipment used and the test methodology employed. Each laboratory should establish its own range of normal values for the particular methods used in that laboratory.

APPENDIX A

Normal blood values— hematology

	Canine	Feline	Equine	Bovine	Ovine	Caprine	Porcine
RBC ($\times 10^6$/µl)	6-9	5-10	6.2-13	5-8	8-15	8-17	5-8
WBC ($\times 10^3$/µl)	6-15	5-19	5-13	4-12	4-12	4-13	10-22
PCV (%)	38-55	30-45	32-57	26-42	24-45	20-38	32-50
Hgb (g/dl)	12-18	10-15	10.5-18	8-14	8-16	8-14	10-16
MCV (fl)	60-77	39-55	34-58	40-60	23-48	16-25	50-67
MCH (pg)	13-25	13-20	14-18	11-17	8-12	5-8	17-21
MCHC (g/dl)	31-36	30-36	31-37	26-34	29-35	28-34	30-34
Neut.segs (%)	60-75	35-75	35-75	15-45	10-30	30-48	28-47
Neut.bands (%)	0-4	0-2	0-2	0-1	0-2	0-2	0-5
Eosinophils (%)	2-10	2-10	1-10	2-15	1-8	3-8	1-11
Basophils (%)	0-.5	0-.5	0-3	0-2	0-3	0-2	0-2
Lymphocytes (%)	12-30	20-55	20-60	48-27	40-75	50-70	39-60
Monocytes (%)	3-9	1-4	0-10	2-7	1-5	1-4	2-10
ESR	5-25 mm/ hour	7-23 mm/ hour	15-38 mm/ 20 minutes	2-4 mm/ day	3-8 mm/ day	2-2.5 mm/ day	1-14 mm/ hour
Reticulocytes (%)	0-1.5	0-1	0	0	0	0	0-2

Normal blood values— coagulation

	Canine	Feline	Equine	Bovine
Thrombocytes × 10³/μl	200-500	300-800	100-350	100-600
Thrombin time (seconds)	4-10	10-19	9-10.5	7.8-9.5
Prothrombin time (seconds)	9-14	10-21	9-12	18-28
PTT (seconds)	17-30	10-25	50-65	37-57
Fibrinogen (mg/dl)	200-400	100-300	100-400	300-700
Bleeding time (minutes)	Buccal 1.4-4.5	Oral mucosa 1.4-2.4	Dermal neck 2.2-3.4	—
Whole Blood Clotting Time				
Lee White (minutes)	5.9-6.3	8.9-9.5	11-13.6	19-21.8
Cap. Tube (minutes)	1-5	1-5.5	3-6	9-10

Normal blood values— chemistry

	Canine	Feline	Equine	Bovine	Ovine	Caprine	Porcine
Total protein (g/dl)	5.4-7.7	5.7-7.6	5.4-7.9	6.0-7.5	6.0-7.9	6.4-7.9	7.9-8.9
Albumin (g/dl)	2.5-4.2	2.2-3.5	2.5-3.9	2.5-4.0	2.7-3.9	2.7-3.9	1.8-3.3
Alk.Phos. (IU/l)	3-16	2-7	11-31	0-38	5-30	7-30	9-31
ALT (IU/l)	4.8-24	1.7-14	1-6.7	4-11	10-12	7-24	9-17
AST (IU/l)	6.2-43	6.7-11	58-94	15-34	68-90	43-132	8.2-21.6
SDH (IU)	—	—	0-2	0-4	—	—	—
LDH (IU/l)	10-36	16-79	41-104	176-365	60-111	31-99	96-160
BUN (mg/dl)	8-28	13-33	10-25	10-25	10-30	10-30	10-30
Creatinine (mg/dl)	.5-1.5	.8-1.9	1-2	1-2	1-2	1-2	1-2
Glucose (mg/dl)	70-110	70-110	75-115	45-75	50-80	50-75	85-150
Amylase (IU)	185-700	280-1800	—	—	—	—	—
Lipase (IU)	13-200	0-83	—	—	—	—	—
Calcium (m/Eq/l)	4.2-5.6	4.1-4.6	5.6-6.7	4.7-6.1	5.7-6.1	5.1-5.4	5.5-5.7
Ttl Bili (mg/dl)	.07-.61	0-.3	0-6.0	.01-.5	0-.39	0-.01	0-.6
Dir Bili (mg/dl)	.06-.12	—	0-.4	.01-.4	0-.27	—	0-.3
Sodium (mEq/l)	141-155	143-156	132-146	132-152	142-150	142-155	110-154
Potassium (mEq/l)	3.9-5.2	3.2-5.2	3-5	3.5-5.1	4.5-5.1	3.5-6.7	3.5-5.5
Chloride (mEq/l)	95-120	105-125	99-109	94-111	103-110	99-110	90-106

Normal values— urinalysis

	Canine	Feline	Equine	Bovine
Specific gravity	1.001-1.070	1.001-1.080	1.001-1.070	1.001-1.045
pH	5.5-7.5	5.5-7.5	7.5-8.5	7.5-8.5
Color	Straw yellow	Straw yellow	Dark yellow	Dark yellow
Clarity	Clear	Clear	Clear to cloudy	Clear
Calcium	2.1	3.0		
Chloride				
Bilirubin	0-trace	0	0	0
Sediment:				
WBC #/HPF	0-5	0-5	0-5	0-5
RBC #/HPF	0-5	0-5	0-5	0-5
Casts #/LPF	0	0	0	0

Blood, Urobilinogen, Glucose, Ketones, Protein—these parameters should be negative for all species.

APPENDIX E

Selected SI units and conversion factors

Constituent	Conventional unit	× Conversion factor	= SI Unit
Albumin	g/dl	10	g/L
Alk.Phos.	IU/L	1	U/L
Amylase	Somogyi units	1.85	U/l
Bilirubin	mg/dl	17.1	μmol/L
Calcium	mEq/l	.5	mmol/L
	mg/dl	.25	mmol/L
Chloride	mEq/L	1.00	mmol/L
Creatinine	mg/dl	88.4	μmol/L
Glucose	mg/dl	.055	mmol/L
Hemoglobin	g/dl	10	g/L
	g/dl		mg/L
Lipase	Cherry-Crandall units	278	U/L
Potassium	mEq/l	1	mmol/L
Protein, Ttl	g/dl	10	g/L
Sodium	mEq/l	1	mmol/L
Transferases	IU/l	1	U/L
Urea Nitrogen	mg/dl	.357	mmol/L

Index

A

Acanthocytes, 56
Acid phosphatase assays for liver function, 110
Activated clotting time (ACT) test in hemostatic evaluations, 77
Activated partial thromboplastin time (APTT) test in hemostatic evaluations, 78-79
Agglutination tests in immune response measurement, 91-92, *94*
Agranulocytes, 28-29, 29-30
Alanine amino transferase (ALT) assays for liver function, 110
Albumin in liver function tests, 105
Albustix protein test, 129-130
Alkaline phosphatase (AP) assays for liver function, 110
Allergic reactions, 90
Amylase, serum, in pancreatic function tests, 114
Anaphylactic reactions, 90
Anaplasma species in blood, 60
Anisocytosis, 54, 55*t*
Antibody structure, 86, *87*, 88
Antibody titers in immune response measurement, 96
Anticoagulants
   for blood samples, 35-36
   oxalate, leukocyte morphology and, 59
Antigen-antibody interactions, 88
Anulocytes, 56
Arginase assays for liver function, 111
Aspartate amino transferase (AST) assays for liver function, 110-111
Autoagglutination, 57
Automated analyzers, 13-14, *15*

B

Babesia species in blood, 60-61
Bacteria
   cells of, in urine, 135
   urine tests for, 132
Band cells, 62
Barr bodies, 59
Basket cells, 62
Basophilia, punctate, 58
Bile acids, serum, measurement of, 107
Bilirubin
   testing for, in liver function evaluation, 105-107
   urine tests for, 131
Bleeding time tests in hemostatic evaluations, 76